Table of Contents

DISCLAIMER

This book is designed to provide information and motivation to our readers. The ideas, concepts and opinions expressed in the book are for general information purposes only.

The information given here is designed to help you make educated decisions about your health and it is not intended as a substitute for any treatment that may have been prescribed to you by your doctor. This book does not take into account your individual health, medical, physical or emotional situation or needs.

For this reason, this book is not designed nor meant to be used as medical advice, nor diagnose or treat any medical condition, nor take the place of proper medical advice from a fully qualified medical practitioner. For diagnosis or treatment of any medical problem, please consult your own physician.

Therefore you should, before you act or use any of this information, consider the appropriateness of this information having regard to your own personal situation and needs. You are responsible for consulting a suitable medical professional before using any of the information or materials contained in this book or accessed through our website, before trying any treatment or taking any course of action that may directly or indirectly affect your health or wellbeing.

The information shared here is the sole expression and opinion of its author based on personal life experience. References are provided for informational purposes only and do not constitute endorsement of any websites or other sources. Readers should be aware that the websites and links listed in this book may change.

The United States Health Department has not evaluated the statements contained on www.eleonoracbastos.com or in any Eleonora Calcada Bastos material.

For the full disclaimer, please see end of the book.

PREFACE

Hi there! And welcome to your very own health journey.

My name is Eleonora and I am a certified health and lifestyle coach.

The reason I decided to become a health and wellness expert is because growing up, after facing a couple of traumatic experiences, I began to suffer with depression and eating disorders. Since I was too young to understand what was really behind my feelings and insecurities, I became obsessive with food and how I looked, as it was the only thing I thought I could control.

I grew up in Milan, Italy, one of the world's fashion capitals, where skinny is the only way to be if you want to be worthy of any attention. So I developed an unhealthy obsession with being skinny, and began to struggle with **negative body image**, which opened the doors to eight years of hell, bouncing from anorexia, to binge-eating, to bulimia. One moment I was starving, then I would binge, then I would throw up 'my guilt' and then 'make it up' by starving myself again and working out like a maniac. I was so disconnected from my body that I used to spend hours staring at it and measuring it, hating every inch of it. It took me eight years to realize I had a problem.

My journey back to health began when I moved to Miami and met Jill, a model, who was creating a brand to deliver a powerful message to women: it's not about starving yourself; it's about making healthier choices. Under her loving guidance, I began healing my relationship with my body and with food. She helped me understand the power of food and the impact it has on our minds and thoughts. Once I started eating 'real food', I immediately felt better, reached a healthy weight, recovered from depression, and started thinking straight. Only then did I finally realize that I was in charge of my life and I was the only one who could change anything. I became passionate about personal development and studied to become a coach so I could share what I have learned and make a difference in other people's lives. Today, I help women all over the world reach balance in their lives through private and group coaching.

In writing Go Feed Yourself, my hope is that it will inspire you to take the first steps towards a healthier lifestyle, finding your own truth. So it's time to get to work. Enjoy!

Love,

E.

SPECIAL THANKS

I want to take the time to thank a couple of people.

Mom, thank you for always supporting me and pushing me forward. I would not be where I am, nor half the woman I am today without your love and guidance. You are the only one who always believed in me every step of the way, even when I did not believe in myself. Although you didn't always agree with my choices, you never let go of my hand and you never fail to encourage me to move forward. You give me hope and strength when I feel lost and defeated. You are my rock and I will be forever grateful to you for everything you have done and still do for me.

Dad, thank you for raising us as independent adults from when we were young, for opening our minds to self-awareness from an early age and for teaching us that anything is possible if we put our minds to it. "Reach for the stars and never settle for less" are words I still live by to this day. Also, thank you for nurturing my passion for personal development, for all the time invested in sharing your advice and point of view, but mostly, thank you for being present in my life.

Bro, thank you to have put in the work that allowed us to get closer than ever and thank you for coming to the rescue whenever I need you. I love you very much and I am grateful to have you in my life.

Jill and Alain, you both supported me during one of the most challenging times in my life, guided me through the process and taught me so much. Thank you both.

Jill, you set me free from my demons. There are no words to describe what that has meant for me and how it has changed my life. Only you know how much you have impacted me with your constant love, guidance and support. It's also thanks to you that I became stronger than ever. You constantly push me to strive to become a better version of myself, to work harder, and want more. You will always have a special place in my heart because of that.

Alain, you are the one who helped me get in touch with my true self. You taught me the power to ask the right questions to control my mind, notice my thoughts, and find the truth that lies behind every emotion. It's thanks to you and Jill that I have become so self-aware and it's one of the greatest gifts I could ever have received.

Marce, you were the first one who supported me in this journey. Thank you for allowing me the freedom to discover and pursue my passion. I will be forever grateful.

I'd like also to thank my tribe of girls, new and old ones. Thank you for always being there for me and making me feel so loved and supported.

And last but not least my partner Morné. Thank you for showing me what it means to be loved unconditionally and be a team. It is the most fulfilling feeling to be in such a strong relationship, where love, support, trust and respect are the foundation of it all. Most of all, thank you for pushing me to pursue my dream and for supporting me in my mission to change as many lives as possible. This book would not have been published if it weren't for your encouragement and support, so thank you from the bottom of my heart.

INTRODUCTION

In the past ten years, the 'health industry' has become a multi-billion-dollar business. Since then, so much research and information has been published on the topics of food, nutrition, exercise and health, much of which is contradictory.

We live in a world where we are constantly influenced in our decision-making by clever marketing techniques. Marketing has become so advanced that even if you think you are strong, you are 'different' and you make your own decisions, the truth is that you are constantly told what to eat, how to look, dress, exercise, sleep, de-stress and so forth, and you don't even realize it.

For this reason, it has become almost impossible to understand and follow what you should eat and do for your health to keep up with the latest and greatest discovery. And how do you find out if the information is there to benefit you or to try to sell you?

That's why I've written this book: to bring clarity and inspire you to **take charge of your own health**.

It was a few years into my coaching practice when I realized how much damage all this contradictory information has done. Besides a general lack of knowledge about food, nutrition and exercise, I have noticed there is also a lot of confusion about what is really healthy and what a healthy lifestyle even looks like. In fact, what I don't like about most programs and health advocates out there is that they support a specific way of eating, training and behaving. They make people believe that to be healthy you need to follow a specific diet plan, work out like a crazy person, have a tight ass, sculpted abs, eat kale all day and do yoga 15 times a week. Well, let me tell you right now: that's bullshit!

So if, at some point, you have felt lost, or still do feel lost and don't know what to eat anymore, what exercise routine to follow and what supplements you should take, don't worry. It's completely normal. And I don't blame you. I was there myself only a few years back and I am here now to help you shine a light on it all.

From my personal journey, I have learned that being healthy is *not* about looking a certain way, following a specific diet or training like a maniac. That's the good news. Being healthy is about having balance and feeling good in your body *and* mind. What that looks like is different for each one of us, which is why we can't follow one plan. We are all unique human beings with different needs, living different lives. What works for one person may be dangerous or even toxic for someone else.

So, how do you get healthy? Well, it's both simple and not easy: you have to reconnect with yourself, which is exactly the goal of this book. In *Go Feed Yourself: The Essential Guide to Feeling Healthier and Happier in Your Body*, you will notice that it's *not* about a set diet plan or workout routine. Rather, this book is a manual intended to hand you all the tools you need to learn how to listen to your body and decode its unique signals so you can finally break free from all the confusion created by following contradictory information and theories on dieting, and start feeling (and looking) amazing in the skin you are in.

To do this, the first part of the book will address your **mindset**, which is usually the biggest obstacle of any sustained change. We have all heard the phrase "you are what you eat," but nobody ever connected the dots: that you tend to eat your feelings and emotions. When you are sad and lonely, you may look for carbs or chocolate. And that is no coincidence!

Once we uncover what areas of your life need work, we will then explore your negative beliefs and replace them with new ones. In the mind section, I will also share some facts with the intention of helping you shift out of the diet mentality once for all.

Once the mind is on board for the transformation, the second part of the book addresses all things *nutrition*. Understanding the basics of food is the single-most important area of knowledge you need to gain in order to make a lasting impact on your life, not just your body, weight and health. Think about it. The food you eat is broken down in your stomach to feed your cells, organs and everything else that your body needs to function properly. If you eat food that lacks nutrients or is loaded with sugars and chemicals, you cannot expect to feel or look good as a result.

In this part of the book, I will pass along simple-yet-powerful facts about certain foods and nutrients with no ulterior motive other than to spread knowledge about food. Together, we will experiment with crowding out the most common triggers of inflammation from what you put in your body. I will also share with you little tricks to help speed up the detox process and assist your body with its natural self-healing process.

By educating yourself about what you put in your body, and by experimenting with it, you will understand the impact that some of the choices you have been making up to now have had on your mind, body, health and weight.

Lastly, the third part of the book shares the **lifestyle shifts** and routines I have implemented in my everyday life throughout the years that allowed me to break free from dieting myself. These shifts have also impacted and improved the lives of many of my clients.

By the end of the book, I hope to have inspired you enough to continue a life-long journey of discovery towards health. *Go Feed Yourself: The Essential Guide to Feeling Healthier and Happier in Your Body* is meant as a starting point for you to learn continually, experiment and discover **what truly works for you**, following your own instincts, not only with food but in life!

It's time to forget about diets and crazy exercise routines. Get ready to reach your body's perfect shape effortlessly! As you embark on this exciting journey towards a healthier you, I encourage you to approach this book as a gift to yourself, rather than 'another attempt to lose weight', so you can finally feel great in the skin you are in.

HOW TO USE THIS BOOK

The idea is that you treat this book as a 12-week coaching program and work through week by week. You will pick a day of the week that you would like to start and that you know works for your schedule. For example: if you pick Monday, every Monday for the next 12 weeks you will **read one full chapter**, so Monday 1 read Week 1, Monday 2 read Week 2, etc.

As several studies have suggested time and again, 12 weeks is the minimum amount of time required to form new habits that will last a lifetime. By the end of the 12 chapters of this book, therefore, you will have found out new information about your body and mind. It is my hope that you will continue this journey of self-discovery on your own thereafter.

At the end of each chapter, you will find some suggestions under the heading TRY. These are simple ideas you can test out or try to implement in your life in a comfortable way to assist your body in becoming healthier in the specific topic covered in that chapter. The suggestions are completely invitational, but they are meant to be implemented into your lifestyle on the day that you read them as much as possible. By working with clients, I've learned that it takes at least a week to feel the effects of giving up a toxic food or substance and to get to the other side of any withdrawal symptoms you might have. That's why it's important for you to implement the suggestions right away on the day you read them; if you decide to follow this book as planned, you will likely start to feel better by the beginning of the next chapter.

At the beginning of each chapter, starting from Chapter 3, you will be prompted to fill out a quick questionnaire to check in with your body and see how you are feeling.

This questionnaire was designed to help you understand how the changes you made the prior week impacted you, if at all, so you can learn what works for your body. This will also help you track your progress, so if you ever lose your motivation, you can look back over the previous weeks and see how far you have come.

PLEASE REMEMBER: Although the book has been designed to last 12 weeks (with the respective chapters timed to be a week apart), follow whatever is right for you. Again, *we are all different*, with unique genetics and health issues, so it is important that you go at your own pace, as the detox process will look different for you than it will for someone else.

It can also be beneficial to remove certain triggers foods for longer than a week to experience the benefits fully. In fact, if you decide to continue removing the foods that you notice are irritating your body for a few weeks more, you will give your body a better chance to tame the inflammation response and focus on healing.

LASTLY: It is possible that you don't think something applies to you as you are reading the chapter title. Or you may think: "There is *no way* I am cutting that out." Rather than skipping the whole topic, I invite you to take the time to read through the chapter regardless, as it may contain new important information that you weren't aware of before. It may not be the case that you need to eliminate it, so please try to keep an open mind and read it through to the end before you decide.

At the end of the book, you will also find a bonus chapter with natural remedies for everyday life situations and a list of my favorite healthy snacks.

HEALTH CHECK: HOW POLLUTED ARE YOU?

When I first moved to the States from Italy, besides adding a good 15lbs to my regular weight within two months, I struggled with many health issues that I had never had before, from chronic fatigue to allergies, dandruff, IBS, acid reflux, the list goes on. It was only when I changed my eating regime drastically that I was able to get my health back on track.

NOT SO FUN FACT: When your body is inflamed, it will hold onto fat for dear life. Inflammation controls our lives. Unfortunately, if you live in the US or the United Kingdom, you are in one of the countries with the highest inflammation among their population. In fact, in a study conducted in 2014, nearly 60% of Americans had at least one chronic condition, 42% had more than one and 12% of adults had five or more chronic conditions[i]. To blame is the Standard American Diet (also named the SAD diet), which is high in pro-inflammatory foods and lacking in antioxidants and other nutrients that help prevent and control inflammation. Unfortunately, the United Kingdom is not so much better either. An alarming study conducted in 2018 by Professor Carlos Monteiro of Sao Paulo University found the British diet to be the unhealthiest diet in the whole of Europe due to its high concentration of ultra-processed 'junk' food such as crisps, chicken nuggets and poor-quality ready-made meals, which now make up just over half of the meals consumed in the average household. Furthermore, the World Health Organization found British people to be the third unhealthiest population in Europe.

But let's take it back for a second. What is inflammation and why should you care? Inflammation is your body's normal response to injury, irritation or infection. It's a process that neutralizes harmful microorganisms, helps repair wounds, and cleans up the debris resulting from the injury. It's something we can often see: the swollen sprained ankle, the infected cut that turns red and tender to the touch and so forth. This is usually a natural and healthy process but it is disastrous when it becomes chronic.

Some of your body's most common signals that it is trying to fight inflammation are:

- Redness
- Headaches
- Allergies
- Food allergies
- Swelling
- Joint pain
- Joint stiffness
- Fever
- Chills
- Fatigue
- Loss of energy/feeling depleted
- Loss of appetite
- Mood swings
- Depression
- Anger
- Muscle stiffness/pain
- Bloating, belching, passing gas
- Diarrhea or constipation
- Fatigue, sluggishness
- Itchy ears or eyes
- Dark circles or bags under eyes
- Joint pain or stiffness
- Throat tickle, irritation or coughing
- Stuffy nose, sinus trouble, excessive mucus
- Acne, cysts, hives or rashes
- Ruddy, inflamed-looking skin
- Flushing
- Water retention, skin puffiness
- Food cravings

- Compulsive or binge-eating
- Heartburn
- Foul-smelling stools
- Sleep problems
- Difficulty concentrating
- Food cravings
- Water retention
- Trouble losing weight
- Skin problems
- Canker sores
- Acne
- Menstrual problems like heavy bleeding, cramps, PMS, menopausal symptoms, mood changes and hot flashes
- Other menstrual disorders
- Bad breath

All of these symptoms are your body's response to a poor diet, toxins and mental stressors. The worst part is that after years and years of toxic overload and suppressing your body's natural detoxing cycle, your major organs will simply give up and stop fighting, resulting in chronic inflammation. Inflammation becomes chronic when it remains an underlying low-level response, creating a constant supply of free radicals that overwhelms our antioxidant defenses and damage our DNA.

This is when we age too quickly and get seriously ill. Some of the diseases caused by chronic inflammation are:

- Alzheimer's
- Anemia
- Asthma
- Arthritis
- Autism
- Autoimmune diseases
- ADD and ADHD
- Bursitis
- Carpal tunnel syndrome
- Celiac
- Chronic fatigue syndrome
- Crohn's disease

- Cancer
- Cervicitis
- Colitis
- Cystitis
- Congestive heart failure
- Depression and other mood disorders
- Diabetes
- Digestive diseases including Crohn's, ulcers, colitis
- Dementia
- Eczema
- Fibromyalgia
- Fibrosis
- Gallbladder disease
- Gastritis
- Rheumatoid arthritis
- Heart disease
- Hepatitis
- Infections
- Insomnia
- MS
- Myocarditis
- Nephritis
- Neuritis
- Osteoporosis
- Parkinson's disease
- Psoriasis
- Prostatitis
- Sinusitis
- Tendonitis
- Vaginitis

When your immune system is too busy to fight off bad food, stress, toxins, allergens, overgrowth of bad bugs in your gut, along with other low-grade infections, your body cannot properly detox. Hopefully, you are not at this stage yet, but if you are, it's okay. In most cases, chronic inflammation is reversible if you are 100% committed to getting better and make detoxification your regular practice.

Helping your body to remove toxins on a daily basis is always a good idea, especially for people with autoimmune conditions. With *Go Feed Yourself*, you will focus on smothering the fire of inflammation that has been secretly sabotaging your weight loss efforts. By the end of this program, you will have all the tools to prevent and reverse inflammation. This will get you a long way towards slowing the aging process, keeping you healthy, young and beautiful for a lifetime.

Are you ready for this journey? It's almost time to start.

BUT BEFORE WE BEGIN...

As I mentioned before, I encourage you to embark on this journey of self-discovery with the goal of freeing your mind and life, rather than another attempt to lose weight, but it's even more than that. Losing the extra weight will happen automatically once you learn how to feel good in your body and provide it with what it needs, but it should not be your main focus while reading this.

After years of struggling with depression and eating disorders, I have finally reached a healthy, happy, fulfilled and balanced life. For me, this means having reached my perfect body weight, feeling full of energy and never getting sick, all while feeling free to enjoy life to its fullest without feeling guilty for any of my choices at any time. My body will look more or less toned depending on how much I work out, but I have been consistent with my weight for six years now — without even thinking about it – yet never feeling like I have missed out in life. I have not counted calories in years, I choose whatever food makes me feel good and happy, I eat out, go to dinner parties, treat myself with chocolate and work out a few times a week — and skip workouts if I feel tired — without **ever** feeling bad about it.

To achieve this level of freedom, the most important thing you need to realize is that we are all unique human beings and that no one body is like another. This means what works for one person may be detrimental for someone else's health and happiness, yours included. In short, you must learn to **tune in** to find what works for you. This is why I am not the kind of health and lifestyle coach who advocates for any particular way of living. I might advise clients to eat less of certain foods or to replace certain behaviors because of the impact on their health, but ultimately I **do not believe in restrictions** of any kind. Personally, I do not follow any specific diet or restrict myself to any specific way of eating. In fact, I would not recommend anyone do so unless they choose to because they truly feel good about it (and not because they are trying to lose weight).

So, the goal of *Go Feed Yourself* is to hand you the tools to learn to listen to your body and create a lifestyle that is suitable for you (your routines and your likings) so that you will feel healthier, happier and more balanced.

I hope you enjoy it!

CHECK-IN QUESTIONS

Before getting into the weekly learning, I'd like to go over some simple questions to assess your current status. The goal of this questionnaire is to help you think with more precision and clarity about your diet and how you feel in your body right now. Then throughout the program, starting at Chapter 3, I will ask you a few specific questions to help you tune in with your body. Then you'll repeat this questionnaire at the end of the book.

Here we go:

Eating habits

Do you indulge in binge-eating or drinking?

Do you eat/snack compulsively or mindlessly?

Do you have cravings?

Are you overweight?

Are you underweight?

Energy level

Do you feel fatigued or sluggish?

Do you feel apathetic or lethargic?

Do you feel hyperactive?

Do you feel restless?

Do you have trouble concentrating or brain fog?

Do you find it difficult to make decisions?

Emotions

Do you suffer with mood swings?

Do you ever feel anxious, fearful, or nervous?

Are you angry, aggressive, or irritable?

Are you depressed?

General health

Do you feel physically weak?

Do you have bad breath?

Do you go to the bathroom regularly?

Do you have acne?

Do you ever have nausea?

Do you suffer with diarrhea?

Do you suffer with constipation?

Do you feel bloated?

Do you frequently burp or pass gas?

Do you have heartburn?

Do you have stomach or intestinal pain?

Do you get hives, rashes, or patches of dry skin?

Do you suffer from flushing or hot flashes?

Are you excessively sweaty?

Are your eyes itchy or watery?

Are your eyelids swollen, sticky, or reddened?

Do you have bags or dark circles under your eyes?

Have you ever had blurry or tunnel vision?

Do you experience ringing in your ears?

Do you have sinus problems?

Do you suffer from hay fever?

Do you have sneezing attacks?

Do you frequently feel the need to clear your throat?

Do you have a sore throat, hoarseness, or loss of voice?

Are your lips, tongue, or gums swollen or discolored?

Do you suffer with canker sores?

Do you ever experience an irregular or skipped heartbeat?

Do you ever experience chest pain?

Do you suffer from asthma or bronchitis?

Do you have shortness of breath?

Do you have difficulty breathing?

Do you get sick frequently?

Do you feel the need to urinate urgently or frequently?

Do you suffer from any genital itch or discharge?

Do you have pain or aches in your muscles and joints?

Do you feel stiff or limited in your movements?

Do you ever feel like fainting?

Do you suffer with headaches?

Do you ever feel dizzy?

Do you suffer from insomnia?

Make sure you reply to these questions in writing so at the end of our journey together you can come back and see how far you have come.

Now that you know where you are, let's dive in.

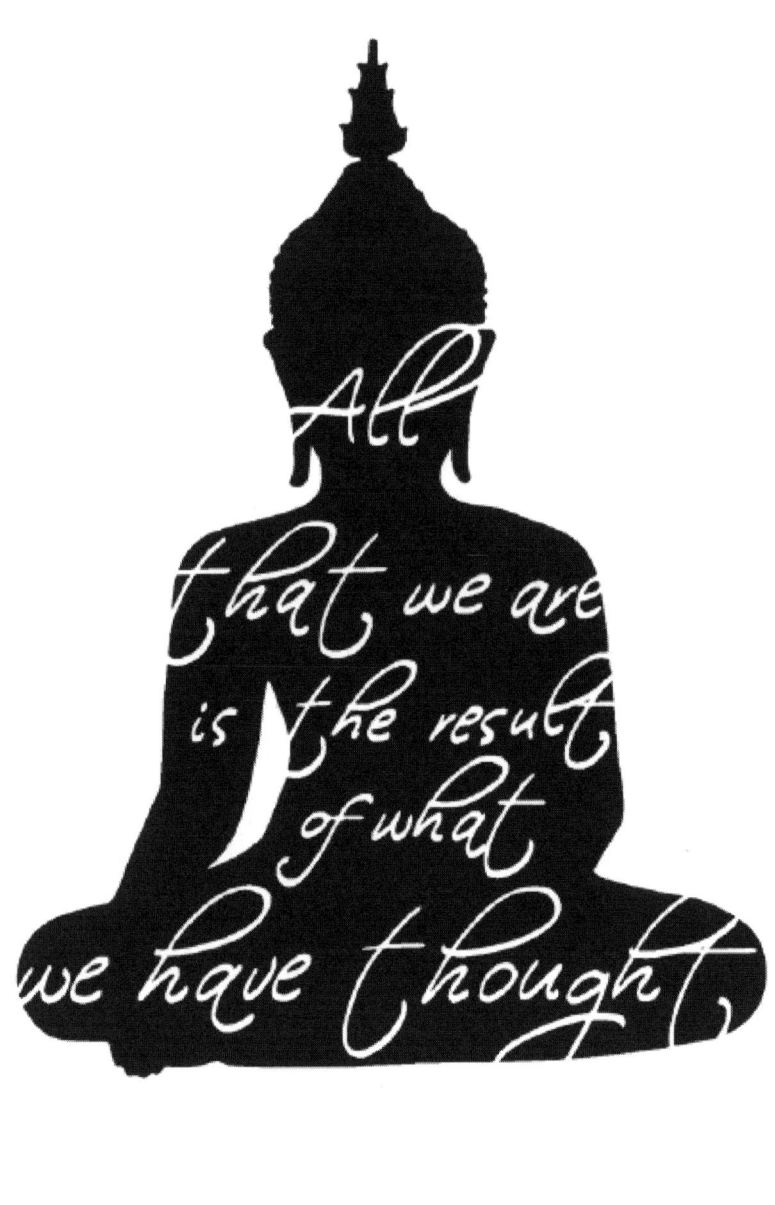

Part

ONE

ADDRESSING THE MIND

Being healthy seems to be the latest trend. Everywhere you look, from magazines to newspapers, from TV to Instagram, you will find girls in bikinis, working out, eating kale and making smoothies, all promoting a 'healthy lifestyle'. And although these can all be great for your health, most of what you see is there to try to sell to you, but they are all missing a huge part of the health picture. I'll get there in a second, but first let me ask you this: Have you ever stopped to think what it actually means to be healthy?

Pause and give this some serious thought. I have asked this question in a number of training sessions that I've delivered and what I find interesting is that people usually attribute the thought of being healthy to a physical condition like eating healthy foods, being fit, muscular or free of disease.

Let me tell you now that there is way more to it. As I explained at the beginning of this book, your emotional health can affect your physical health and vice versa. This is what many people refer to as the infamous **mind-body connection**.

In fact, you can eat all the kale in the world, take your vitamins, drink water and work out consistently, but if you don't deal with what's inside of you (and by that I mean in your heart), you will still be unhealthy.

What I mean by that is that in order for you to be in good health, you have to live a balanced life. This means paying attention not only to your body and nutrition, but also to all areas of your life, including your love life, your career, your family, your finances, your relationships and friendships, your spirituality and so forth. Allow me to explain why.

Your feelings, emotions and social wellbeing are just as important a component of your overall health as nutrition and workout regimens. In fact, our physical bodies react to our mental or emotional wellbeing just as much as to our nutrition. This means that every feeling you have affects some part of your body and can wreak havoc on your physical health. So even if you're doing everything 'right' with your nutrition, your emotions — both chronic and acute — can still ruin your body, causing aches, pains and even disease. (There is so much to say about this that it could be a whole other book). For now, trust me when I say that detoxing your mind, heart and spirit is just as important as detoxing your body.

The problem with this is it's not so easy. Unfortunately, we live in a society where we are persuaded and brainwashed spiritually, emotionally and mentally on a daily basis, which is what brought us to completely lose touch with ourselves and our uniqueness. If you think about it, since you were born, you have been conditioned to be or act a certain way: from your parents to your teachers, from your friends to the media. You were taught that everyone's opinion is important. And before you knew it, you were bombarded with information on how you should look, act, think or speak in order to be accepted.

We are hyper-hypnotized every day to produce, consume and press on without questioning the system. In this high-speed society, where we are constantly bombarded with information and technologies, our lives are buzzing with all kinds of obligations and distractions, leaving many feeling empty and lost. These standards — although often unrealistic — slowly became our reality and (rightfully) we lose ourselves in the process ending up unable to deal with this world.

As such, the first step towards becoming healthy is to address your mental and emotional wellbeing. This means it's time for you to take responsibility for your needs and desires, develop an intimate connection with your body and mind, and let go of all your preconceived notions about what is right or wrong. It's time for you to grant yourself the entitlement to be happy and allow yourself to discover and nurture your own unique self.

What is *your* definition of freedom and happiness? Is it the life that you are living or is there a little voice inside you that says there has to be more to life than this?

With that, I encourage you to take responsibility for your own health and happiness. Find your truth, listen to your body's needs and desires, and develop a great understanding of your body, mind and soul so that you can thrive in life. Begin to play with life once more. Try something new, dance uninhibitedly, change jobs or switch careers, take risks and discover yourself!

Without any more delay, let's get started with the very first step, getting your mind aligned!

*"I like to
avoid things
that make me fat...
...like scales,
mirrors and
photographs"*

WEEK 1

BRING YOUR MIND ON BOARD

If you, like me, have ever tried to make lifestyle changes, you know that the biggest obstacle to overcome is your mind. In fact, it is your mindset that usually sabotages your progress by making excuses, setting unrealistic expectations, putting pressure on yourself, talking you down, minimizing your results and so forth. But here's the thing: *No lifestyle change will ever be successful if it only focuses on your body without addressing the mind.*

This was one of the biggest revelations I ever had. After years of trying any diet I could think of and being stuck between eating disorders, I was finally able to break free from dieting, never count another calorie again and simply enjoy food.

What changed? My mindset. But more so, my beliefs.

So, the first step of our journey together is dedicated to addressing your mind so it can support you on your journey of self-discovery.

First things first. You need to get your foundations right. That means uncovering your beliefs about yourself, getting perspective on what's 'true', then completely detaching from unhelpful beliefs to move forward and never go back.

Week 1 will help you do exactly that! Get ready to **un-become** everything you have learned to be and turn into a brave explorer, ready to create a new path with your own steps, rules and dreams. It takes courage to thrive in a society that isn't always set up to support your values, interests, and beliefs. Get ready!

UNCOVERING YOUR STORY

Each one of us has a story — or many — that shaped our life. I have mine, you have yours and your friends have theirs. At its core, your story is where you live emotionally, mentally, and sometimes even physically. Your story can either be the fuel that keeps you going or the ball and chain that weighs you down.

At some point in life, we all go through something that *shouldn't have happened to us*. For the most part, that something happened a long time ago. So, while it's important to recognize what events and experiences have made you who you are today, you cannot expect to move forward if you're holding onto your entire life's baggage. It would be like trying to go for a run while chained to a 500lb weight.

Just imagine what your life would look like if you felt great in your body and were full of hope, inspiration and vitality, like nothing bad had ever happened to you.

HOW TO UNCOVER YOUR STORY

I know, I know. This is way easier said than done. It took me a great amount of work to learn how to do it, but here's the good news: I did it and I am now here to teach you how to do it too… and in a much simpler way.

In order to flush out self-limiting beliefs, first you need to identify them. This exercise is not meant to make you feel bad or self-conscious about your past, but is aimed at helping you identify the roadblocks so you can move forward once for all. We all tell ourselves stories about why we don't do something or can't achieve what we want, so know you're not alone.

To start identifying the beliefs, stop for a moment and ask yourself why you have not yet achieved your health goal. What is the belief or series of beliefs that stop you achieving good health or great physical shape? Make sure you don't filter the responses. Write down everything that comes to mind. No excuses, no rationalizations, no going into denial. Everything that comes up needs to go on this list. If nothing comes to mind, usually it means that there is a 'valid excuse' or a belief on why you have not achieved what you wanted. What is the story in your head?

Now, when you have a list (even if it's only one item), think about where that belief comes from and write next to each belief what made you believe that. Usually, beliefs come from outside interactions, such as a parent, a teacher, a partner, TV, social media, and almost never just you on your own. It's important to identify whom they came from so you understand that your beliefs were not yours (in most cases) but handed to you.

When you have identified them, not only can you understand that unhelpful beliefs and excuses are not true, but you are able to reverse them and replace them with new empowering beliefs that propel you toward reaching your goals.

Take the time to think how these beliefs have negatively impacted your life.

Did these beliefs lower your self-esteem?

Did they make you angry, sad or lonely?

Did they make you isolate yourself?

Did they leave you with doubts or confusion?

Did they make you fearful?

Did you need to see a therapist for them?

Did they cost your health?

What about your relationships?

Did you lose someone you loved in your life because of that?

What about your career or performance?

Did these beliefs prevent you from being or becoming who you wanted to be?

What about your peace of mind?

Chances are that you have answered 'yes' to one or more of these questions. If so, it's time to assess and write down how much it cost you. What loss have you suffered or problems have you developed because of these beliefs? Don't worry about writing full sentences. Just as long as you can clearly see everything you lost because of them.

Now think to the future and really recognize how these beliefs could affect you in five to ten years from now. What would you miss out on because of these beliefs? Recognize what they have cost you and will continue to cost you if you don't change. Is this really what you want?

SAY IT OUT LOUD

Before you get started on this activity, please know that this exercise is not aimed at minimizing your experiences in any way, shape or form. What I am asking you to do is try to gain a new perspective and look at your difficulties as relative when comparing them with other people's 'success stories', especially if those people endured the same or worse as you and are now some of the most powerful people in the world. Nobody in this world has ever lived without challenges. It's absolutely impossible. Challenges are part of life. There is nothing wrong with that. But what is wrong is the way that we process what has happened to us.

Keep in mind a lot of successful people you may know have endured unthinkable cruelties (beating, rape, torture, war, etc.) and tragedies (homelessness, losing a body part, losing a loved one, and so forth), yet they are now entrepreneurs, role models and business people. Take, for example, Tony Robbins (grew up poor and escaped with brother and sister at 17 to protect them from alcoholic mother), Richard Branson (has dyslexia), Oprah Winfrey (lost her child), Kris Carr (overcame cancer), Jim Carrey (was homeless), Charlize Theron (witnessed her mom kill her dad), to name a few. These people succeeded because they overcame their dark pasts, refused to let tragedy and hardship define them, and created a new story using their past experience as fuel for change.

One way to get rid of your story is simply to say it out loud and listen to how silly it sounds. Try saying, "I don't have a good life because…" or "I cannot reach my goals because…" Go back to your list and say each belief or excuse out loud, several times, over and over again.

In my own life specifically, my excuses were: "I don't have a good life because I was sexually abused" and "I cannot reach my goals because nobody gets me." Obviously, certain times in my life were pretty traumatic and I hope you did not have to endure the kind of pain I did, but if you have, then please know there is a way out.

More common stories can be: "I cannot reach my goals, because I'll have to spend time with certain people" or "I cannot reach my goals, because I don't have time" or "I cannot reach my goals, because no one will love me if I'm too successful."

Yes, it's embarrassing, but that's the point. Your story may have been upsetting (even traumatizing) in the past, but when you say it out loud as an adult, you will hear how limiting it is. Repeat each story aloud until it starts to sound silly. When you become disgusted enough or exhausted enough with the old limiting story and you feel ready to replace it, come up with a new one.

LOOK FOR THE GOOD

I was the victim of my story for so long that I learned to subconsciously look at every difficulty in my life as stuff happening **to** me. I would ask myself all the time, "Why is this happening to me?" One of the biggest mindset shifts that changed my life for the better happened when I was challenged by one of my mentors to shift out the victim mentality and look for the positive in my story.

When you learn to approach life as though adversity is happening **for** you and not **to** you, you can stop suffering under all the things that bother you.

Every person on this planet at some point had to endure something unfair or tragic. Unfortunately, nothing can change the past and the pain you may have experienced up to this point. But every experience is here to serve you. Pain helps you grow, mistakes help you learn and losses help you gain; ultimately, they all force you to evolve. The direction you evolve in is entirely up to you. You can spiral down and let them take over, detracting from your life. Or you can choose to see the good that the situation created in your life as it helped you blossom and become who you were meant to be.

So, imagining life happens **for** you, how does that shift in perspective change your outlook? What does it do to the stories that you have built up that very likely tear you down and hold you back? In other words, if there is a lesson to be learned with every adversity, you just need to learn to recognize and accept it. If you think about the situation with hindsight, there is always something better in store. Every experience gets you exactly where you need to be. That's how you got right here.

Although things might not always go as you plan, if you remind yourself that everything is happening for your greater good, you will be able to breathe through it and live more easily and happily.

I know this is easier said than done, especially when you are going through stuff and still in pain. I have to remind myself about this constantly, even now, but if you can remember this and make it a mantra for life, you will feel free and uplifted knowing that you might face challenges, but their happening is part of a bigger plan.

MANTRA: *"This is happening for me. It's taking me exactly where I'm supposed to be. I trust that something better is coming."*

Make a conscious choice to perceive challenges as something beneficial so that you can deal with them in the most productive way.

FLIP YOUR STORY

Now it's time to flip your limiting story and turn it into an empowering one. Here's how to do that. Search the internet for proof of people who have gone through the same as you but have overcome it and become successful. Go out and seek the proof that shows you it's possible to get out of your current situation. Find their story, get inspired and create your own.

If what happened to you happened **for** you, what is the good that came out of it? And if you could have anything you wanted, what would you want to achieve?

Type it into your phone, write it on a piece of paper, or email it. How you do it doesn't matter, as long as you write it down and take a couple of days to think about and perfect your new beneficial story. Once you've created it, keep it somewhere that you can read it every single day for the next 12 weeks. Read it in the morning and before going to bed. And not only read it, but read it out loud. This is really important, so please make sure you do it this way, because you have programmed your brain for 10, 20, 30 years or more, and this is the most effective way to reprogram it. Speak your new story out loud. Let the vibrations run through your body and see how that feels. Find a friend who would understand and appreciate hearing your new story and speak it aloud to them. Ask them to hold you accountable. All they need to do is remind you of your story when you're slipping back into your old patterns.

You have spent so many years with your old story that it can take some time to erase it, so just be consistent and patient. Commit to repeating it every morning and evening for the next 12 weeks and watch the results unfold.

From now on, focus on the present moment, leaving all past experiences, preconceptions and judgments behind you. There's no point in keep dragging your past into your present. It will do you no good and it will only limit your future. What is past is past. You can learn from it but you cannot change it, so why waste your time dwelling on it?

MOVING FORWARD

"If you don't know where you are going, you will end up elsewhere." — Laurence J Peter

Now that you have uncovered your past, it's time to do some strategic planning. First, you will assess which areas of your life need attention. Then you will set goals for this journey together. And lastly, you'll take a look at some strategic planning and imprinting to make sure that when the journey gets a little tough, you can come back for some motivation.

WHEEL OF LIFE

"The first step for change is awareness." — Nathaniel Branden

It's now time to bring awareness to your current situation, so you can consciously understand what is missing (or not working) in your life, take control, and start creating the life of your dreams! As we saw at the beginning of this book, being healthy also means feeling good emotionally, which is why we cannot address your physical body alone. The Wheel of Life exercise looks at the main areas of your life that are responsible for your physical and emotional wellbeing. It is one of my favorite tools to help quickly and graphically identify the life areas that need a little more attention. As weird as it may sound, all these areas in life play an important role in becoming healthy and happy, and as such, losing the extra weight for good. Why? Because you cannot pretend to make any lasting change in your nutrition, unless you feel good about yourself and your life. The only way to do that is to address what is going on inside of you. So let's get started.

How to use the Wheel of Life tool:

In the next page you will see what the Wheel of Life look like. There is a scoring system behind using the Wheel, where you simply reflect and rate your satisfaction levels out of 10. The center of the circle is to indicate complete ***dissatisfaction*** with life; the perimeter is to indicate complete ***satisfaction*** with life.

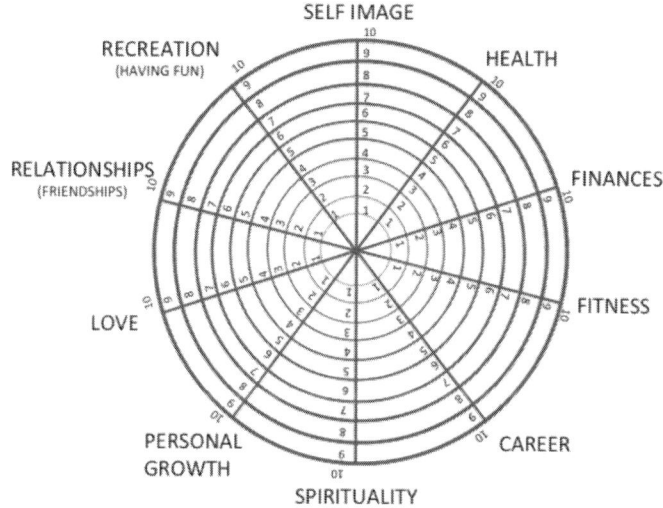

Follow these easy steps:

1. For each category, place a dot along the white line to indicate how satisfied you are with that life area. Use a scale from 0 (completely dissatisfied) in the center to 10 (completely satisfied at the edge). See example below.

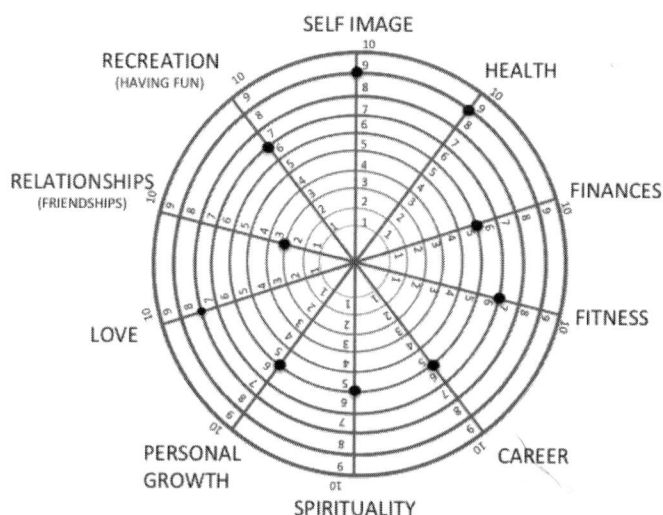

2. Connect the dots to see your circle of life.

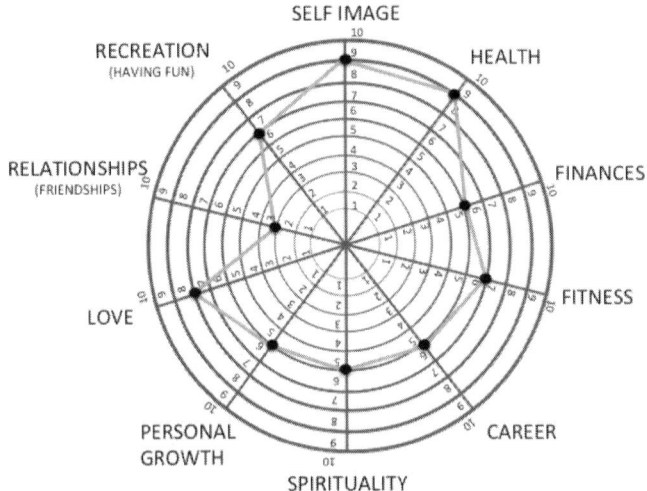

3. Now that you have a visual representation of your current life balance and your ideal life balance, identify the gaps. These are the areas of your life that need your attention.

4. Try it yourself! Grab a pen and fill out the first empty diagram as directed.

You will notice that there are almost certainly areas in your life that are not getting as much attention as you'd like. However, there may also be areas where you're putting in more effort than you need, sapping energy and enthusiasm that may be better directed elsewhere.

A balanced life does not mean scoring 10 in each area. Everyone is different, but the goal is to score a minimum of 6 in each life category. A happy medium flow.

SETTING REALISTIC GOALS

Now that you have identified what areas need work, it's time to plan the actions needed to regain balance. Setting goals is an extremely important step in achieving what you want. But before you do that, it's super important that we spend a few moments on the importance of setting *attainable* goals. Why is this so important? Because the only way the plan will work is if you set goals that you know you can accomplish. Having high expectations and ending up disappointed is one of the main reasons why people stop going after what they want.

- **Be as specific as possible**

  For instance, consider what resources you need to make it happen, how much it will take, how expensive it will be, and so on.

- **Think about the limitations**

  Every goal also comes with aspects that can potentially stop you from achieving it. In order to make sure you're being realistic, consider all the limitations you might encounter while trying to achieve your goal.

- **Make sure you're fully committed**

  One of the biggest mistakes people make when setting goals is not fully committing to achieving them. If you truly want to succeed, you have to feel it deeply in your heart. When imagining the outcome, if it's not a hell yes, then it's a no, and you should focus on something else instead.

IMPORTANT: When I coach clients, we usually implement just one or two new habits per week, because if you commit to too many things, you end up committing to nothing. This is why I would recommend that you focus your attention over the next 11 weeks on addressing just the Self Image section of the Wheel of Life.

Remember, your mind is the biggest obstacle to overcome here, so if you set unrealistic goals, you are setting up yourself for failure!

YOUR BODY'S PERFECT SHAPE

If you have bought this book, I imagine there is something about your body you would like to change. So before we get any further with setting goals, we need to address the way your body looks in your eyes.

What do you think of your body? What thoughts or words come to your mind? Do you find yourself stressing out, getting sad or feeling anxious because you don't look like the girls on social media?

It has been estimated that 90% of women say that their body image causes them to feel down. And worst, a recent survey[ii] found that on average, women have 13 negative body thoughts daily. This means that the average woman has nearly one negative thought about their appearance every waking hour. A disturbing number of women confessed to having 35, 50 or even 100 hateful thoughts about their own shapes every single day.

If you find yourself agreeing as you read this, know that the unrealistic standard of beauty that our current society portrays has affected you. But it's not your fault and it's completely normal — as you can see. I have suffered with this myself. Despite overcoming most of my negative body demons years back, I still need to pay attention to my thoughts every now and then. In fact, as a woman approaching my 30s, I have to admit there are times I still catch myself looking at other women in my industry or 'models' on Instagram and wish my body was that flawless or my hair looked that shiny and bouncy. Sometimes, I even caught myself questioning my authority because I don't look like some of my colleagues, which is pretty damn scary if you think about it. Luckily, I have learned to snap out those thoughts quickly. But if you think that those images have the ability to influence a grown woman like me — even if it's just for a second — what can it do to young girls who are still growing, developing and discovering who they are?

Yes, we all want to look attractive and there is nothing wrong with that. The problem is what we have come to view as 'average' or 'normal', which is an unrealistic idea of youth, thinness and beauty. In fact, we live in an era where digital and physical alteration has become the norm. The use of filters, special cameras, professional make-up and lights has created an idea of beauty that is **unattainable in real life**. The extensive use of digital touch-ups — not only limited to TV and magazines like back in the day — has created standards that are seriously damaging our body image and the way we view ourselves.

FIGHTING THE TREND

Every person struggles to become fully comfortable in his or her skin, but worse than this is the fact that research suggests women who obsess over their body and diet have chronically elevated levels of the stress hormone cortisol. Too much cortisol in your body can suppress your immune system and cause blood sugar imbalance, diabetes, weight gain, obesity, cardiovascular problems, infertility, thyroid problems, dementia, insomnia and other conditions. That's why it is so important that you learn to get a hold of your negative thoughts in general, but especially the ones related to your body.

So, how can you shift out of this unhealthy state of mind, created by these societal trends? When I first moved to Miami, I was still suffering body dysmorphia and eating disorders, so I decided to attend a seminar to try to overcome my negative thoughts. Miami is a melting pot of cultures and we were a group of 20 women from all over the world. There was this one exercise that stuck with me, where the presenters made all the participants sit in a circle around a drawn female figure. One by one, we had to draw on the figurine (each one of us with a different color marker) what the 'perfect woman' looks like in our culture. It was really interesting to see that we had completely different — if not opposite — visions of what 'perfection' looked like. That's when it struck me: Perfection does not exist.

We create an ideal and call it perfection, but it is merely a decision, our decision. We decide what perfect looks like, influenced by our culture and upbringing. In fact, beauty ideals change over the years and differ completely between countries. The idea of a perfect body is different from person to person based on when and where we form our beliefs, so the reality is that there is no perfect body at all.

In 2015, a UK online pharmacy (Superdrug) created a project called *Perceptions Of Perfection* with the goal of showing how much the 'perfect body' varies depending on geographic location, proving once again that such perfection is imagined and does not exist in reality. For this project, the company hired 18 female graphic designers from countries around the world and gave them a stock image of a woman and asked them to Photoshop the image to reflect the beauty standards of their specific countries. You can see more about it if you search 'project perceptions of perfection'.

So, now that you know that the perfect body does not exist, the next most important step — one that has helped me heal my relationship with my body — is to learn and understand the different body shapes.

WHAT'S *YOUR* BODY SHAPE?

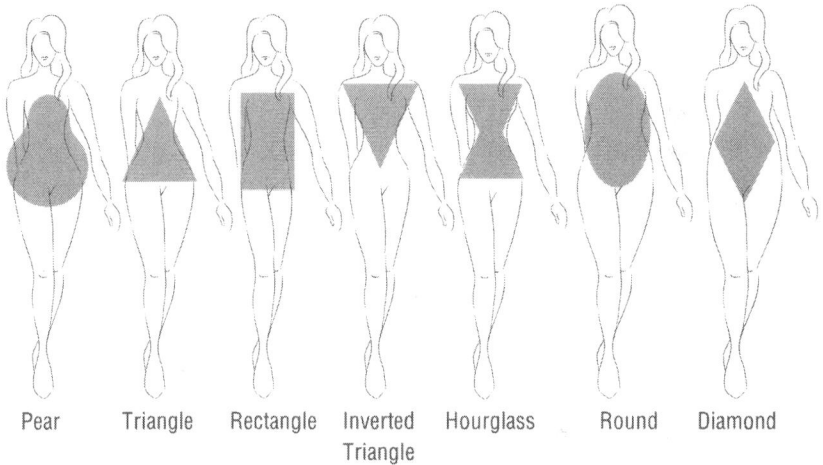

Pear   Triangle   Rectangle   Inverted Triangle   Hourglass   Round   Diamond

There are seven different body types in women:

- **Pear:** Pears have larger lower bodies and smaller upper bodies — storing fat on the hips, thighs and butt. You have an elegant neck and proportionately slim arms and shoulders. Your waist is your best asset so don't be afraid to show it off.

- **Triangle:** Your hips are larger than the bust and have a 'shelf' appearance. Your waist is slightly smaller than the bust. You are prone to gaining weight in your tummy and have a tendency towards love-handles.

You may gain weight in your upper thighs and upper arms, but your lower legs and arms are your best assets.

- **Straight:** Also called *rectangle* or *ruler* body shape, this is the most common body type. Over 45% of American women have a straight body shape. Your hips and bust are balanced but your waist is not very defined. You probably have a bottom that is more flat than round and you tend to gain weight in your torso first and then your upper thighs and arms.

- **Inverted Triangle**: Also known as an *athletic* body type, you have a proportionally larger upper body, with broad shoulders, ample bust and a wide back. Your hips are slim and your bottom may tend towards the flat side. You have a tendency to gain weight around your belly and in the upper body.

- **Hourglass:** Your bust and hips are well-balanced and you have a defined waist. You also have gently rounded shoulders that align with your hips. You most likely have a rounded bottom and your upper body is proportionate in length to your legs.

- **Round:** Also known as the *apple* body shape, you have a large bust, narrow hips, and a full midsection. You have a tendency to gain weight in your stomach, back and upper body. Your waist is undefined and the widest part of your frame. You also have a full, shorter neck, a full face and your buttocks are somewhat flat with slender legs. Legs are your best asset.

- **Diamond:** As rare as its name, your hips are broader than your bust and shoulders, and you have a tendency to gain weight on your stomach, back, hips and buttocks. Your waist is undefined and the widest part of your body. You have proportionately slender, shapely arms.

Now that you know your individualized body shape, here is how you fight the trend. First of all, you need to understand something: **you will not be able to change your body's shape**. It's a waste of your time and energy. I can tell you this from experience. Learn from my mistakes: I am a pear shape, tending to hourglass (curvy with a big butt), but for the longest time I wanted my body to look like a model, which is usually a rectangle shape and flat. I have starved myself to the extreme and worked out obsessively trying to reach that shape. The result? Even once I reached my lowest weight ever (99lbs — and I'm 5'7" tall, so yikes!), my body's shape remained the same.

So instead, the goal is to **achieve your body's best shape**. Instead of focusing on weight loss or transforming your body's figure, which is not possible, the best thing you can do for yourself is to aim to be fit, healthy and happy, so you can look in the mirror and appreciate what you see.

Lastly, you need to **shift your thoughts.** Beauty is just as much about how you feel about your body as it is about how you look. Truth is that beauty comes in all shapes and sizes; even the most beautiful and confident women have insecurities sometimes. The only difference is that they have learned to combat those thoughts, rather than allow them to take over. That means learning to rewire your brain, which is worth it, not just your peace of mind, but your *physical* health as well.

BOTTOM LINE: Finding the sweet spot means aiming for your body's *natural weight and shape*, where you don't have to restrict and get paranoid about what you eat or how much you work out, and then learn to accept it as it is.

You don't have to adhere to what the media portrays as 'perfect', whether you're a man or a woman. If you want a more toned physique or simply to look better for yourself, that's fine, but remember the most important thing is to be happy and healthy while achieving it. You don't have to go to the gym every single day, unless you decide to go because it makes you happy. Provided you are fit and healthy, there's nothing wrong with not having a six-pack or perfect legs. Happiness and balance are way more important than sporting a sculpted figure just to be recognized by our twisted society.

Being healthy and happy begins with body positivity. Loving your body starts with taking care of it. Starving yourself on a low-calorie diet or exercising obsessively isn't the way to go. Eat well, take care of yourself and maintain an active lifestyle. If you follow these simple principles, your body will achieve its best shape effortlessly and you will boost your confidence, as well as feeling a hell of a lot better.

Focus on achieving your body's best shape and start seeing your body for what it really is: a beautiful, diverse, flawed, amazing, resilient thing that allows you to do so much. There's no perfection in this world, just different point of views. So choose yours wisely.

TAKING ACTION!

It's now time to put everything you have learned into action. First, you will answer some questions on why are you here today and then you will set goals based on your Wheel of Life.

I encourage you to not just answer the following questions in your head, but to **write them down**. Maybe you can even copy these answers down somewhere so that you can always have them with you for easier access.

WHY ARE YOU DOING THIS PROGRAM? *Are you here for weight loss? Are you trying to resolve a health issue or getting rid of bad eating habits? Do you just want to learn more about food? What made you buy this book?*

_____

_____

_____

WHO ARE YOU DOING THIS FOR? *Are you doing this for your self-esteem? Because you just want to feel better? Or for your partner, family or friends? Understanding the why behind your goals will bring clarity and help you stay focused.*

_____

_____

_____

WHAT BELIEFS OR FEARS ARE HOLDING YOU BACK? *For example, you may fear failure (or failing again), you think losing weight is too complicated or you don't think you deserve to be in shape. What is your excuse not to do this?*

_____

_____

HOW DOES YOUR CURRENT SITUATION AFFECT YOUR LIFE? *Look at your current state of health as well as the current state of your relationships and think about your overall life goals.*

WHAT WILL YOU ACHIEVE IF YOU REACH YOUR GOAL? *What benefits do you hope to gain and how will your life change?*

Now let's look at your Wheel of Life results. I recommend choosing to work only on the Self Image area for the next few weeks together, the reason being, if you choose too many things to do, you will likely feel overwhelmed, which will increase your chances of failing. You are here because there is something within you in relation to your body that is not working for you, so let's focus on that for a start. Once you finish the 12 weeks, you can come back to this exercise and address a different area.

Here are the questions.

WHAT ARE THREE SPECIFIC ACTIONS YOU CAN TAKE TO REGAIN BALANCE? *For example, what can you stop doing, reprioritize or delegate to someone else?*

_____

_____

_____

WHAT ARE THE TOP THREE THINGS THAT COULD HOLD YOU BACK FROM MAKING THESE CHANGES? *The more obstacles you can bring to light, the better chance you have of navigating around them.*

_____

_____

_____

HOW MIGHT YOUR LIFE BE DIFFERENT IF YOU SUCCEED?

_____

_____

_____

Make a commitment to these actions by writing them down, because doing the exercise in your head does not have the same effect.

Now that you have a clearer idea on what your goals and obstacles are, you have a better chance of navigating around them. In the following weeks, if you ever lose your motivation, come back to this part of the book and read the answers you gave to the above questions to remind yourself why you are doing this. Pick yourself up, brush yourself off, put on your big girl panties and rock this new lifestyle!

GOODBYE CHEAT, HELLO TREAT!

Let's get one thing straight. I don't believe in cheat days or cheat meals. You're here because you want to learn how to live a healthy life. And guess what. Living a healthy lifestyle **doesn't mean restricting yourself** or missing out! After all, everyone loves pizza, pasta, maybe a cupcake every once in a while… As my mom would say, indulgences are good for the soul.

Now, read over the following sentence until it really sinks in:

One bad meal will not undo your progress.

Read it again.

One bad meal will not undo your progress.

Cheat meals or cheat days are not about the foods we eat, but the mentality that surrounds these terms. The words we use have a powerful effect on our brain, body chemistry and mood. When addressing a meal or a day as somehow cheating, the stress response around doing something 'bad' is oftentimes unhealthier than the food choice itself. This is why I think the whole concept of 'cheat meals' needs to be dropped, because of the negative connotations around the word 'cheat'. For this reason, I'd like you to make a conscious change from this point forward around the way you perceive and talk about a not-so-healthy choice.

We are human and humans love to treat ourselves every once in a while. Instead of viewing a not-so-healthy choice as something 'wrong', where you stuff your face and feel guilty right after, learn to enjoy your treat as something truly worthwhile. From this point on, let's call your not-so-healthy choices a 'treat' rather than a 'cheat'. Doesn't it feel much better already?

A relaxed approach to slip-ups will make you much more likely to succeed with your new lifestyle. When you are treating yourself with something delicious, here are four of my best suggestions:

Always try to pick the healthiest version possible of whatever you are going for. For example, if you want to go for a brownie, don't get the processed pre-packaged one. Rather, bake your own, maybe replacing the ingredients with the best quality ones or go to a bakery and get the freshly homemade version.

Try to limit treats to a couple of times a week. One not-so-healthy choice will not undo your progress, as long as you don't declare a whole day a treat day!

Make sure you hydrate well an hour or two after a treat meal and try to walk afterwards. I am not suggesting doing a workout. Just a simple 15-minute walk after your treat will help your body flush out toxins and help your digestion process.

When you can, try skipping the extra dressing, condiments, topping or frosting. Eat the same amount you would regularly (if not less) but enjoy the s*** out of it. For example, instead of eating a cupcake 'as is', scrape out the majority of the frosting and leave only a thin layer. It's a small adjustment that will make a big difference.

If you learn to let go of the fear that one not-so-healthy meal will reverse your progress, you free yourself from the stress reaction that could actually have worse effects on your weight than the choice itself.

OVERCOMING COMMON EXCUSES

Everyone struggles with excuses. It's part of our human nature. The problem with excuses is that they keep us from getting results or making changes. With proper motivation, you could and would make anything happen. For example, if I were to give you $1 million to read this book and follow it to the letter, you would make it happen. You see, most of the time, we create excuses just because it's hard to make a change. We get lazy or we get scared. It takes a lot of effort and guts to stand out from the crowd, but starting to work on your integrity (actually doing what you say you're going to do) will help you on so many levels.

Here's a rundown of the most common excuses and how to overcome them once to help you adjust your perspective.

The "I DON'T HAVE ENOUGH TIME" Excuse

I know you're busy, but so am I and so is everyone else on this planet. But eating well isn't as time-consuming as you might think. It's all about planning your meals smartly, so you can stay on track.

Let me give you an example. If you're always running out the door in the morning, choose a breakfast you can prepare the night before. Another trick I like to use is to prepare a batch of quinoa, millet or rice on a Sunday night, so I can use it the whole week as a base for all my meals. Get creative and make it fun.

The "HEALTHY FOOD IS BORING AND TASTES LIKE CRAP" Excuse

This was one of my biggest misconceptions about healthy food. But guess what. It's not true. Not even close. If what you have tried so far doesn't taste good, it's time to look for better recipes.

Take a peek at the recipes on my website or get your butt on Google and start looking for new stuff.

Also keep in mind that your taste buds will change and adjust over time, so after a few weeks, you might find yourself appreciating the foods you are currently trashing.

The "HEALTHY EATING IS EXPENSIVE" Excuse

Eating healthy food *can* be expensive. I get that. Especially if you have a big family to take care of, it can come at a price. But not eating healthily will cost you even more in doctors' bills and medicine! If you don't have the budget to afford a complete makeover, here are a few tricks that could help.

Replace your most frequent foods with the healthier version: Oftentimes, people will replace what they eat least often with a healthy alternative, rather than what they consume the most often. It should be the other way around! It's what you eat every day that impacts your health, not those sporadic treats or so-called cheat meals.

Check out the EWG Dirty Dozen list: This list is created by a non-profit organization in the US and is updated every year.

The foods on this list have the highest levels of chemical contamination. If you buy the conventional version of these foods, it's like eating a chemical bomb, so make sure to buy these ones organic as a priority.

See page 151 for the list.

The "I'LL DO IT LATER" Excuse

You've purchased this book for a reason, so stop procrastinating! Every single day counts. The more you wait, the more you are going to pollute your body and mind, and the further you will drift away from your goals. There will never be a 'right time'. You are living now. So, cheer up and let's make it happen once for all!

Believe in yourself and call out your own BS. If I paid you serious money to make things happen, you would do it, so enough with these excuses! Your health is worth it.

GETTING ACCOUNTABLE

The transition process to a healthier life can be quite overwhelming. I encourage you to seek the help of a certified health and lifestyle coach to help and support you in a fun and empowering way on your journey towards achieving your best health. I know that not everyone has the financial resources to afford a health professional, with programs starting at $150 a month and rising fast, so the next best option is to ask a friend, family member, co-worker or someone in your faith or community to join you on this journey. Here's why.

Often, we see detox as a solitary pursuit, but the truth is that it will be easier if you find a way to integrate your friends and family into the experience. Social support makes a huge difference. Not only will it be more fun, but having support will also help you to stay on track and motivate you when you get discouraged.

Social isolation is toxic in the extreme. In a study published in the Proceedings of the National Academy of Sciences of the United States in 2013, isolation was linked to all causes of mortality among both men and women. You can do everything right — eat, sleep, exercise, and be as 'pure' as possible in your lifestyle — but if you are not connected, you can easily still get ill. As my mentor Joshua Rosenthal would say, "We are spiritual beings in a material world." We hunger for play, touch, validation, spirituality, intimacy and connection just as much as we do food. So, if you can talk a friend or family member into doing this process with you, that's great! You'll enjoy sharing food and good health, as well as having someone to compare feelings with along the way.

Here are a few fun ideas for buddying up:

- Host healthy dinners or happy hours at your house. Make it fun and share what you learn.

- Find a walking buddy. Taking a friend with you on a short walk reinforces your commitment to exercise and helps you release stress. Plus, you will have the added bonus of bonding.

- Tell a friend. Even if you can't persuade anyone to join you on your detox journey, find a friend or two to talk to about what you are doing.

ONE LAST THING: If you connect with other people who are committed to the same goal, you'll feel empowered to succeed. Make sure to ***join the online Facebook*** community at www.facebook.com/thedietfreeproject and be present! ***Ask***

lots of questions! This is your chance to learn as much as possible, so you can maintain this lifestyle forever. Someone on the team will be there to answer any doubts or concerns, plus you will be able to get support from other people who are going through or who have gone through the same steps as you're going through now.

Remember, losing weight and getting healthy are social activities! You can do the program alone, but if you find a buddy, join or create a group, or join our online community, it can be easier and more fun!

JOURNALING

A food journal is one of the most important tools for a successful journey to wellness. As adults, we are completely in control of what we place in our mouths, but as our busy lives go on, we tend to eat more than we think we do. We underestimate our daily intake because we fail to take into consideration portion size (usually much larger than we imagine), sometimes graze, and forget about the fluids we consume.

Keeping a food diary will hold you accountable and force you to pay attention to what you are eating. By writing down your experiences, you will reduce stress and learn to connect what you eat with how your body *feels*.

Studies show that tracking your food intake for at least a week will have the best results. If you don't want to carry a pen and paper at all times, you can use the notepad on your phone, rewrite the questions from your journal and type the answers there. Whatever you do, please avoid relying on your memory, as there is a high chance you'll forget something and that could be adding up unnoticed. At first, you should use your food diary to keep track of the meals you eat, but over time you can use this as a tool to plan out basic meals and snacks, paying attention if you're skipping meals or noticing you're not eating enough of certain food groups.

SPECIAL REQUEST: Please be honest with yourself. The purpose of this exercise is to bring awareness to what you are eating and how you are feeling. This tool is made for you to support you, not to put you down. It is a picture of where you are, not where you are going, so please don't lie to yourself or feel judged or ashamed. Remember that you are doing a food diary just for yourself. Being honest and accountable to yourself is crucial for success.

DITCHING THE DIET

Now that we have covered the mind and those potential obstacles, the last step for permanent weight loss is to lose the diet mentality. How many diets have you tried that promised to make you feel good, look better, drop the weight and boost your health? I lost count a long time ago! Throughout the years, I tried a crazy amount of fad diets, only to find out that none of them really work. The faster I made a change, the faster and harder I failed.

I am sure every woman on the planet at some point in life falls into this trap. And men do too. No one is to blame though. When government doctors and food authorities try to promote the same lifestyle "eat less, work out more" and "it's all about dieting and calorie balance," it is hard to believe otherwise.

But is dieting a trap? The global market for weight loss is estimated to be worth $586.3 billion dollars. The problem is that this market is created around setting unrealistic weight loss goals and results so that everyone keeps on dieting. This industry **makes money from failure**, not success, so that you will become a returning customer and pay again and again. Think about it: If you really lost weight for good, you would be a one-time consumer! Not a great business model!

*Dieting is by definition a temporary food plan, based on the notion of **restriction, willpower and control**, which makes it impossible to be a sustainable lifestyle for the rest of your life.*

The deprivation of restrictive diets can lead to overeating or a binge-eating cycle. Not only that, but dieting only tackles the symptom (needing to lose weight) rather than the underlying cause (what's keeping you from being slim), the cause being poor habits around nutrition. What makes this more confusing is that even the worst diet will likely result in some initial weight loss, but **about 95% of people will regain the weight within one to five years**. Most of the time, people put the weight back on after just a few weeks or months. Can you relate? After an unrealistic diet or lifestyle, the vast majority of dieters usually become frustrated and give up. Then, after a few months back in their old pattern — and often back to their initial weight — they feel guilty and get 'back on track' with the latest and greatest fad diet, starting the famous yo-yo process all over again, which brings a lot of health risks along with it.

Studies show that only **5 to 10% of dieters are able to keep the weight off in the long term**, and when they do, it's by devoting every minute of their life trying to fight biology and evolution. After months spent on restrictive calories or fad diets, your body will put up a compensatory mechanism to defend against weight loss by decreasing how much energy you expend (slowing down the metabolism) and increasing appetite (to make up for the lack of energy), which will make it even harder to lose weight. In most cases, this will result in weight gain. People tend to blame this on the dieters 'falling off the wagon' and 'having a lack of willpower', but biological changes are taking control. Are you sure you want to spend every living moment fighting against yourself? My guess is you don't.

So, how can you lose weight for good and let it feel good? As I said before, it's all about finding balance. And I'm not talking about calorie balance!

THE TRUTH BEHIND CALORIE-COUNTING

According to some studies, people who count calories are eight times more likely to develop an eating disorder than people who don't because of failure to reach their weight goal. I was one of them. In fact, I have been a slave to calorie-counting and diets for a third of my life and I can tell you it does not work out well.

It is common for people who want to lose weight to just cut calories; exercise takes a lot of time and effort, and many people don't even enjoy it. You've probably tried cutting calories to lose weight at some point as well. Maybe it even worked. After all, it makes sense. If you use 2,500 calories a day and you eat 2,000 calories, those leftover 500 calories that are needed for your body to function properly have to be burned from somewhere. But the faster you lost weight, the more likely you lost water and muscle, rather than fat.

Why? Remember when I explained that your body put in a compensatory mechanism to prevent sudden weight loss? Well, it happens with calorie restriction as well. You'll eventually reach a 'plateau', a point where the scale refuses to drop any lower, no matter how little you are eating. If you continue to cut your calories by fasting, skipping meals, or starving yourself, you will do terrible damage to your body. In fact, what happens is your body will then begin to eat itself in order to get the nutrients your brain and body need to work properly. That's right. First, your body will grab the water it needs from your water composition. Then, it will start eating up your muscle. Only last will it eat your fat reserves. So, if up to now you have lost weight on a low-calorie diet, it's likely you have not lost fat, but water and muscle, which is why you put it all back on when you started drinking and eating normally again.

And it gets worse! With only a few weeks of deprivation, your immune system will also get weakened and you will become more susceptible to diseases. If you keep on starving yourself, your body will eventually start to get its nutrients from your bones, reducing their density: a true disaster. You deserve better than that!

But why does your body attack the fat last when restricting calories? For your brain to work properly, it needs glucose found in proteins like the ones in your muscles. But let's take a closer look on why calorie-counting does not work.

NOT ALL CALORIES ARE CREATED EQUAL

The vast majority of conventional nutritionists, doctors, government health advisors, the food industry and the media are all still actively promoting the outdated, *scientifically disproven idea* that as long as you burn more calories than you consume, you will lose weight. Let's face it, if that advice was good and doable, we would all be thin and healthy by now. But that notion is simply dead wrong, as not all calories are created equal.

Researchers have found that, in many cases, overweight individuals actually consume approximately the same number of calories as slim people. How is this possible? If it's a matter of calories in versus calories out, how can two individuals consume the **same** number of calories, but one remain thin and one gain weight? The answer is that they are not eating the same kinds of foods.

Let's take it back for a second. **What even is a calorie?** A calorie is the measure of how much 'energy' a food contains. The notion of cutting calories for weight loss was born because of Newton's first law of thermodynamics. I don't want to get into too much detail here. Bottom line is that Newton identified in a laboratory that 1,000 calories of broccoli and 1,000 calories of soda have the same energy amount. This is actually true. The key phrase being 'in a laboratory'. But Newton's law doesn't apply in living digestive systems. The food you eat interacts with your biology, a complex adaptive system that instantly transforms every bite into energy for different functions. Your body doesn't treat all calories the same way.

In fact, do you think your body would **feel** the same after consuming 400 calories of ice cream as it would consuming 400 calories of brown rice and steamed vegetables? What about if you were to eat 400 calories of chocolate donut versus eating 400 calories of baked potato and chicken? When would you feel better? Even a kid could tell you that eating 400 calories of veggies and 400 calories of ice cream is not the same.

One of the reasons why calorie-counting is an obsolete concept is that there are way more factors that play a role in our digestive process besides the calorie amount present in our food: amount of chemicals, sugars and fats to name a few.

CALORIE DENSITY

There is another factor to keep in mind: calorie density. Calorie density measures how many calories are in a given weight of food, as in calories per pound. A food high in calorie density has a high number of calories in a small portion (by weight) of food, whereas a food low in calorie density has far fewer calories in the same weight of food. Therefore, choosing foods with a lower calorie density allows us to consume our usual amount of food (or more) while reducing our caloric intake.

Here's an example:

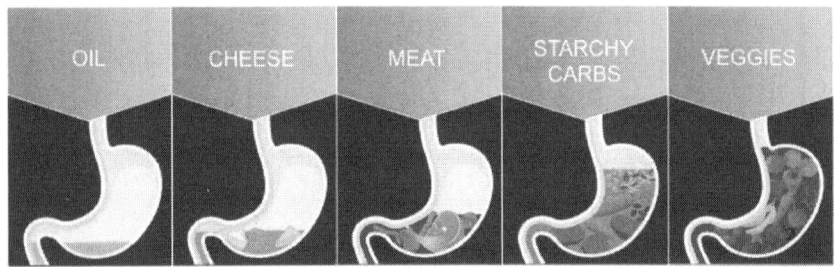

In the image above, you can see how much space 500 calories takes in the stomach. As you can see, you can consume a larger portion of a low calorie density food (whole foods like veggies and potatoes) than a high calorie density food (oil, cheese, etc.) for the same number of calories.

In addition, lower calorie density foods (fruits, veggies, starchy vegetables, intact whole grains and legumes) are also the foods highest in nutrient density. This means that by following a whole food diet, not only you will feel full and satisfied faster, but you will consume fewer calories and more nutrients! So, are whole foods starting to make more sense?

The fact that all calories are not created equal is the single most important thing you need to learn about healthful eating and lifelong weight management. This approach to nutrition will allow you to manage your weight without feeling hungry. By following this simple principle of calorie density, you will also increase the overall nutrient density of your diet.

Understanding the concept of calorie density was one of the most powerful piece of knowledge I learned in order to shift my mindset, fully heal my relationship with food and break free from calorie-counting. Only once I understood this simple concept did I stop counting calories and being scared of food. That's when I shifted my focus from calories and quantities to eating whole, nutrient-rich, high-quality foods until I felt full. When you eat whole, nutrient-rich, high-quality foods, and feed your body with all the nutrients it needs in order to thrive, *you do not even need to count calories*. In fact, when fed properly, your body will feel fuller faster. This will control your appetite, eliminate your cravings and keep you at a healthy weight. I am living proof.

A diet filled with processed foods, added sugar, and refined grains can be more satisfying in the moment, but you will be more likely to overeat, which will prompt your body to store fat. Choose wisely. You deserve that!

So, what are these whole, nutrient-rich, high-quality foods? These include non-starchy vegetables (leafy greens, mushrooms), nutrient-dense proteins (seafood, eggs, grass-fed beef, low-fat plain Greek yogurt), and whole-food fats (avocado, flax seeds, etc.). These foods will fill you up quickly and keep you full for a long time. They also trigger the release of hormones that tell the body to burn fat. One thing they all have in common? You don't need a nutrition label to tell you they're healthy. So, relax about keeping a calorie journal and *focus on the quality* of your food.

PORTION DISTORTION

Now that you understand why you should abandon the diet mentality once for all, our society's biggest problem for achieving good health is portions. Food and drink portions have increased dramatically since the 1980s. Eating the right amount of food is an important part of being healthy (and losing extra weight). Although your parents may have encouraged you to finish all your food when you were younger, this is rarely healthy. The amount we eat is too often dependent on how much we're served. The more on our plate, the more we eat. And bigger portions can cause people to eat 30 to 50% more than they usually would.

Monitoring portion size as well as choosing healthful nutrient-dense foods can make a huge difference in whether you feel great or lack energy. In fact, consuming the right balance of nutrients is really important for the normal functioning of your body, and for fat loss, muscle gain or weight maintenance.

Instead of going crazy measuring your food, which to me sounds very restrictive and unsustainable — because what happens if you go out to eat or you are invited over at a friend's place!? — I have learned a quick and easy way to teach my clients the perfect food composition for each meal. With every meal, you should consume mostly vegetables and proteins with a little fat and some form of carbohydrate.

A helpful simple way to remember portion size is to use your hand as a measuring tool as shown below:

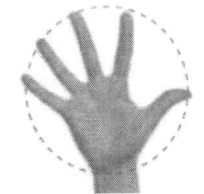

Circumference and thickness of hand spread (or more!)

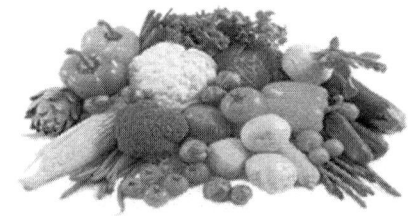

High-water content, whole, fresh fruits and vegetables

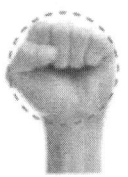

Volume of clenched fist

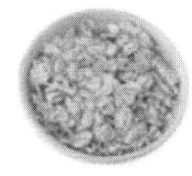

Complex carbs & whole grains • Legumes & vegetable proteins

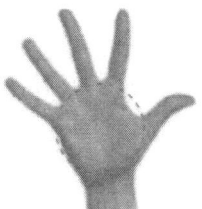

Circumference and thickness of palm

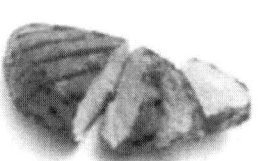

Low-fat animal proteins • Protein-rich nuts & seeds

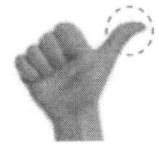

Diameter and thickness of thumb (or less!)

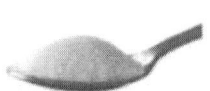
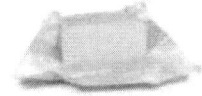

Simple sugars • Dressings & spreads • Desserts

In general, your plate should look as follows:

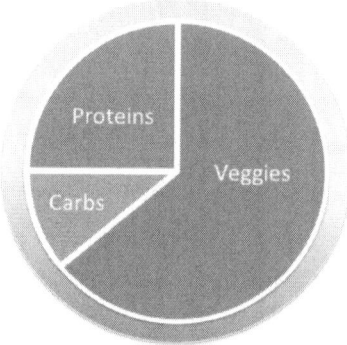

TRY: BALANCED EATING WEEK

Now that you have a clearer idea of calories and good portion sizes, it's time to put your new knowledge into action! This week, you will focus on eating in a more balanced way and remove the stress of calorie-counting. Here's how:

- Make sure you eat a portion of vegetables and protein, a little fat and some form of starch with each meal.

- Vegetables should fill at least half your plate.

- Follow hunger cues! The above recommendations are just a guide, but you should always follow your instincts. Eat more or less based on your appetite, but make sure to keep the proportions the same: mostly vegetables and protein, a little fat and some form of starch. (If you are trying to lose weight, eat carbs only once a day, either for breakfast or lunch. Avoid carbs at dinner.)

- Choose mostly whole foods with minimal processing, unrefined and organic when possible.

- Make sure you're not starving when it's time to eat your main meals. If you are, have a small salad or a glass of water before your meal.

- Have two snacks throughout the day (mid-morning and mid-afternoon). This will keep you satisfied and decrease the urge to eat large portions at traditional mealtimes.

BOTTOM LINE: The corner stone of health is achieving mind-body balance. However, this isn't as simple as it sounds. To achieve balance, you must have complete knowledge of your life. Human beings are so much more than physical bodies; rather we have layers of emotions that play a huge role in our health and wellbeing. We are a result of what we eat, but we tend to make food choices based on our feelings and emotional state, which is why I believe it is impossible to address the physical body without addressing the mind. Don't forget that unprocessed emotions are just as harmful as processed foods; they add heaviness and toxicity in the body. It is essential for you to work through your past to build a brighter future.

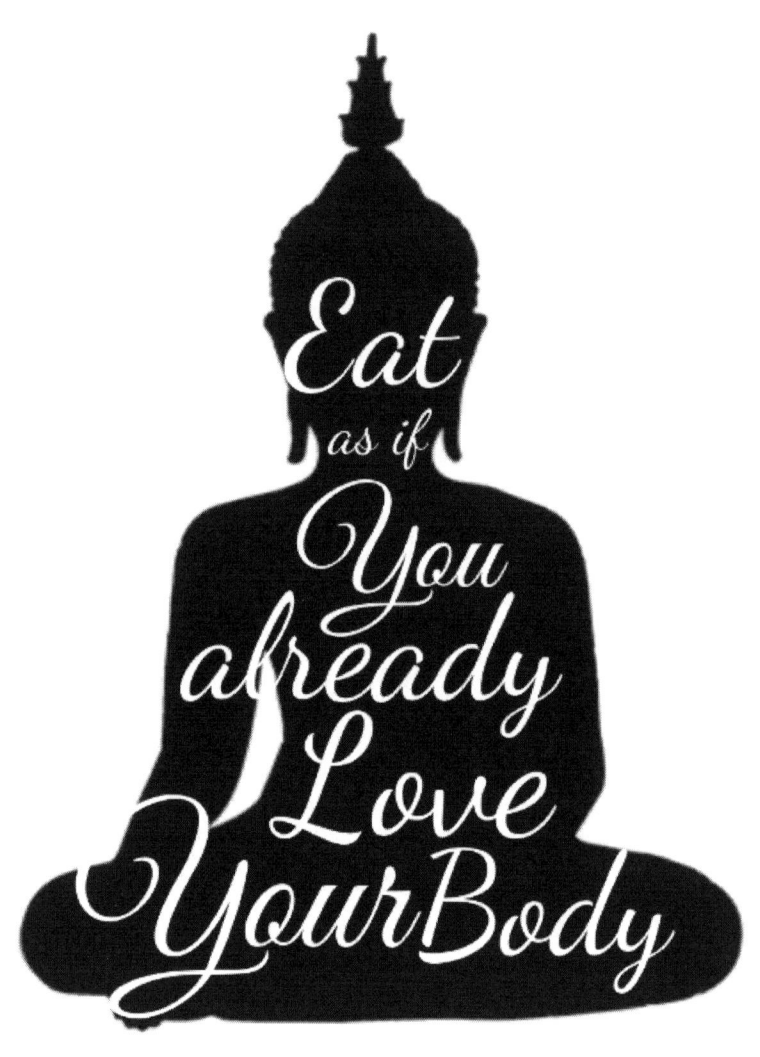

Eat as if You already Love YourBody

Part TWO

ADDRESSING THE BODY

"The mind and body work together. Your body needs to be a good support system for the mind and spirit. If you take care of it, your body can take you wherever you want to go, with the power, strength, energy and vitality you will need to get there." – Jim Rohn

*"I like to take
long romantic walks…
to the fridge…
…or the pantry"*

WEEK 2

PREPARE YOUR BODY

Food is critically important in this process of self-discovery. What you put inside your body is what you get back. What you eat is what creates your cells, tissues, blood, skin, hair... It's also responsible for your mood, your energy levels, the way you feel and even the way you think! Once your diet is in place, everything else will follow magically. I say this from personal experience.

One of the biggest shifts I made was to stop obsessing over how I looked and start focusing on how I *felt* and the quality of my food – what nutrients I was eating rather than how many calories. By doing so, not only did I gain so much freedom in my head, but I reached my body's perfect shape and maintained it effortlessly.

This chapter is meant to help you get clear on some basics of nutrition so you can understand how the food you eat impacts your body and health so that you can make conscious, educated decisions when choosing what to eat. I truly believe that knowledge is power, and that if people understood the power of food, they would make different choices.

SPECIAL REQUEST: Please skip detoxification pills, laxatives, 'fat-burning' pills and all of that. Stop fasting or counting calories for weight loss. Instead, focus on what nutrients you are feeding your body. Seriously, lasting weight loss cannot be obtained by quick fixes like starvation, dieting or magic potions. So, forget all your preconceived notions about healthy eating and follow these steps so that you can discover what works *for you* and create a healthy lifestyle that you can enjoy for the rest of your life.

WATER

Nothing on this planet can survive without water. Aside from oxygen, water is the most-needed nutrient of any living, breathing creature. Humans are just one of the many examples.

Drinking enough water is one of the simplest, most basic and important steps that you can take towards health. Our bodies are made up of approximately 60% water, which means that they need water to function properly. Water helps transport nutrients, increases energy, flushes out toxins, prevents headaches, promotes weight loss, regulates body temperature and much, much more. Dehydration can have profound effects on your health. Common symptoms of mild dehydration are: dry mouth, dry skin, fatigue, lethargy, muscle weakness or cramps, headaches, dizziness, nausea and forgetfulness.

DRINKING ENOUGH OF THE RIGHT KIND OF WATER

So, how can you tell if you are drinking enough water? Depending on your size, your body can only process a bit more than a glass of water per hour. This is one of the main reasons behind the infamous recommendation: drink one glass of water every hour. As a general guideline, you want to drink a minimum of 8 to 10 glasses of filtered water a day.

The easiest way to know if you're hydrated is by checking the color of your pee. Ideally, it should be light yellow or almost clear and should not smell. If you are taking riboflavin (vitamin B2), which is also found in most multivitamins, your urine should be bright yellow, almost fluorescent. If it is a deep yellow, then you are likely not drinking enough water.

Now that you understand the importance of drinking water for your health detox, you're probably thinking that all you have to do is turn on the tap, fill a glass, and get it going. Unfortunately, it's not that simple. Here are a few tips to ensure you won't drink any toxins and do your body a disservice:

Filter your water. Filtering your own water at home is absolutely the best way to ensure its quality. Heavy metals, pesticides, antibiotics and other drugs, disinfectant products, radioactive particles, bacteria, chemicals, mercury, fluoride and arsenic are just a few of the pollutants found in most water supply in the United States. Chlorine, lead and mercury are the most common and all of these chemicals are detrimental to your health; if consumed for a long period of time, they can cause damage to the heart, blood vessels and nervous system, cancer and much more. If you want to know more about these negative health effects, I suggest investigating further what these toxins can do to your body, but in short, these are why it is so important to obtain a water filter for your home and make sure you drink healthy water.

Although there are hundreds of brands of home water filters, they all rely on a small number of technologies to remove contaminants. The three main ones are:

- **Carbon filters:** Pitcher, tap-mounted or large dispenser carbon filters are affordable and can reduce many common water contaminants. Their effectiveness may vary: Some just remove chlorine and improve taste and odor, while others remove a wide range of contaminants including lead, mercury and volatile organic compounds (VOCs). However, activated carbon cannot effectively remove common 'inorganic' pollutants such as arsenic, fluoride, hexavalent chromium, nitrate and perchlorate and will grow bacteria if not replaced as recommended.

- **Reverse osmosis:** The higher initial cost of a reverse-osmosis filter can be well worth it, given that it will remove everything that a carbon filter does, plus MTBE, bacteria, viruses, parasites, arsenic, heavy metals, fluoride, sulfates, nitrates, radioactive particles, and asbestos. These filters can be mounted on countertops or underneath kitchen sinks and work in conjunction with your plumbing system to offer water on demand.

- **Ceramic filter**. Ceramic filters eliminate bacteria, cysts, chlorine, foul tastes and odors, herbicides, and pesticides. Many ceramic filters have silver baked into them, which inhibits the bacterial growth that can be a problem with standard carbon filters.

Avoid bottled water. Industry reports show that up to 44% of bottled water is just regular tap water. Despite the hefty price tag, by purchasing bottled water, you are not necessarily buying better quality. There is also some concern about the types of plastics being used to store water as the plastic additives may migrate from the bottle to the water. About one third of >100 bottled water brands tested for contaminants were found to contain chemicals like arsenic and carcinogenic compounds at levels exceeding state or industry standards. Fluoride is also usually still present in bottled water.

It can be difficult to avoid using plastics, especially when you're trying to up your water intake, but there are a few precautions you can take to avoid drinking toxins in your water:

- **Avoid freezing any bottled water**, as it leads the plastic chemicals to leach into the liquid.

- **Avoid using plastic bottles (or cups) for warm or hot liquids,** or avoid leaving them in the sun or in a warm environment as the heat will have similar effects to freezing.

- **Avoid washing and reusing plastic water bottles,** because by doing so, more chemicals will leach into your water.

- **Do not put your plastic water bottle in the dishwasher**, even if labeled 'dishwasher safe' or 'BPA-free'.

- **Store your water in glass or stainless steel containers**, as these are the best options for drinking water. They can be washed and reused almost indefinitely, and they don't leach any chemicals into the liquid.

- **Refill your own glass bottles at home for daily use.** Not only is this the cheapest option, but it's also less harmful to your health and the environment, because it stops the need for throwaway plastic containers.

- **Avoid purchasing the one-gallon cloudy plastic (PVC) containers** from your grocery store as they transfer far too many chemicals into your water. The five-gallon containers and the clear bottles (polyethylene) are a much better plastic and will not give the water a plastic taste.

Personally, I use a stainless steel or glass water bottle that I can refill at home or at a filtered water fountain at work or at the gym. If this is too much hassle, then please do follow the tips above to avoid harm to your body.

THINK BEFORE YOU DRINK

Flavored water, 'zero calorie' water, 'vitamin' water and so-called 'enhanced' or 'functional' water products have become quite popular lately, especially among the health-conscious. Unfortunately, most of these waters do more harm than good. In fact, many of these water mixes are loaded with fake, chemical additives, including artificial colors, preservatives, and artificial sweeteners, many capable of wreaking havoc on your metabolism, hormones, and other physiological processes. Yikes!

My best suggestion if you really don't want to drink just plain water? Try flavoring your own water with sliced lemons, cucumbers, mint leaves or other fruits, and leave these water substitutes behind. If you need an extra energy boost for your workout, ditch all the chemical-laden sports drinks and use coconut water instead.

DAIRY

Dairy is a controversial topic. Health organizations promote dairy as vital for improved bone health, yet other experts disagree and claim dairy as detrimental to health. Who is correct? I'm going to stay away from the ethical, religious and political aspects for the sake of this argument, and just give you some information so that you can make educated decisions about consuming it, and if you do, how much.

Have you ever stopped to think about how we are the only mammals that drink milk after infancy? What about the fact that we are also the only animals to drink another species' milk? And have you ever thought about how, biologically, cow's milk is meant to feed a rapidly growing calf?

Although we were led to believe that dairy was good for us, truth is it's likely robbing you of better health. If you suffer with any of these, dairy could be the culprit.

- Allergies
- Eczema
- Asthma
- Arthritis
- Bloating
- Gas
- Constipation
- Diarrhea
- Acne
- Fatigue
- Headaches

In fact, over 75% of humans on the planet are unable to properly process milk because they don't produce the lactase enzyme, which is required to break down lactose, a sugar found in milk. Beside this, when we consume milk and its derivative, we are also ingesting antibiotics and growth hormones that are given to cows in order to reduce their risk of illness and maximize production.

I know what you're probably thinking: What about milk being a great source of calcium? Well, dairy actually acidifies the body's pH. When the body's pH becomes too acidic, minerals are 'pulled out' of bones and tissues to compensate, leading to osteoporosis, sarcopenia (muscle loss), fractures and kidney stone formation, possibly diabetes, high blood pressure, heart disease, thyroid problems, cancer and other insidious conditions.

Even if you are not lactose intolerant, dairy can sometimes contribute to bloat, gas and abdominal distention, which no one wants anyways! Additionally, limiting your dairy intake can improve your skin, helping it stay clearer with fewer breakouts.

BOTTOM LINE: Our natural state is to be lactose intolerant. By consuming dairy, you go against your body's nature, causing inflammation, which leads you to battle major health issues down the line. Even though goat's milk and sheep's milk are much easier to tolerate, they have similar lactose content to cow's milk so the effect on your body is the same.

Don't panic though! Luckily for you, there are many milk alternatives on the market right now, like rice milk, almond milk, cashew milk, or coconut milk. Just make sure to read the labels for harmful ingredients or sugars; I always buy the unsweetened versions and make sure they have only a few natural ingredients.

There are also many other great non-dairy sources of calcium, my top 10 being:

- Almonds
- Almond cheese

- Almond, hemp or coconut milk

- Broccoli

- Collard greens

- Figs

- Kale

- Oranges

- Spinach

- Sesame seeds

If you are concerned about your calcium intake, know that the recommended daily dosage is 1,000 mg a day for men and women up to the age of 50, and 1,200 mg per day for people age 50 and over. Since it is hard to reach this daily amount of calcium from foods, I use calcium supplements to help meet the need, not as a replacement for food, but as a way of supplementing my diet. As a general guideline, I never recommend removing an entire food group from someone's diet unless they have a medical reason for doing so. However, a good way to keep dairy in your life *and* lose weight *and* be healthy is to limit your portions and not exceed twice a week. Lastly, if you stick with consuming milk and dairy, try always opting for organic, as it has higher levels of omega 3 fatty acids and CLA, and more antioxidants and vitamins than regular milk; you also avoid any concerns with pesticides, fertilizers, hormones and antibiotics.

CARBS

If you think of your body as a car, then carbohydrates are the fuel. Consuming carbohydrates is important in ensuring the body has what it needs to operate at peak performance.

Now, you may think of carbs as evil because you're imagining foods like pizza, pasta, cookies and so forth. Well, let's get this straight. There are good carbs (complex carbs) and bad carbs (simple carbohydrates). If you're interested in the science behind how they work within your body, you can go ahead and read all about it online, but in this book, I'm going to keep things super simple. Here's what you need to remember: although a little counterintuitive, simple carbs are the processed ones while complex carbs are the ones from nature. Let me explain why.

Simple carbohydrates are refined (processed), which means the natural minerals, vitamins and fiber content are removed. This makes simple carbs a source of quick energy but little nutritious value, which is why they are sometimes referred to as empty calories. Cakes, baked goods, table sugar, candy, fizzy drinks, white bread, sugary drinks, pastries and chocolate bars are your typical refined, simple carbs.

Complex carbohydrates are the good source of carbs, as they come from nature and are rich in fiber, minerals and vitamins, which help slow down the release of energy in a more sustainable way, while feeding us a bunch of good stuff.

So whether you're trying to lose weight or just be healthier, do yourself a favor and try to eliminate sources of simple carbs and indulge in the complex ones. Below is a list of the good guys.

FRUITS

- Raspberries
- Kiwi
- Blueberries
- Pomegranate
- Strawberries
- Apples
- Pears
- Grapefruit
- Prunes

NUTS, SEEDS AND LEGUMES

- Lentils
- Kidney beans
- Chickpeas
- Split peas
- Black beans
- Pinto beans

VEGGIES

- Kale
- Garlic
- Tomatoes
- Onions
- Okra
- Dill pickles
- Carrots
- Yams
- Peas
- Radishes
- Beans
- Broccoli
- Spinach
- Green beans
- Zucchini
- Cucumbers
- Asparagus
- Sweet potatoes
- Plantain
- Parsnips
- Green peas

DAIRY

- Low-fat yogurt
- Milk

WHOLEGRAIN BREADS AND PASTAS

- Breads and pastas made with the whole grains listed below provide more fiber, resulting in feeling fuller sooner and for longer.

- Whole grains
- Buckwheat
- Brown rice
- Corn
- Wheat

- Barley
- Oats
- Sorghum
- Quinoa
- Air-popped popcorn

BOTTOM LINE: The type of carbs we eat can either harm us or help us. Try to eat carbs in their natural form and stay away from refined ones, as they are just bad news.

FATS: THE GOOD, THE BAD AND THE UGLY

Now, let's address another poor part of health that was stigmatized for a long time: fat. Although you might have spent your whole life thinking that you should swerve fat, it is essential to your health and supports many of your essential bodily functions, including energy, healthy hair, skin and nails, vitamin absorption, and others.

Just like calories, not all fats are created equal. There are good kinds of fat and bad kinds of fat. Good fats promote several health benefits such as protection against heart disease, cancer, Alzheimer's, depression as well as reduced blood pressure and lower cholesterol. Bad fats on the other hand increase the risk of diabetes, stroke and heart disease.

The most important thing you need to know is how to recognize good and bad fats. Let's start with the good guys:

GOOD FATS: UNSATURATED (eat these!)

Healthy oils and fats are actually (and ironically) great cleansers. These fats are essential to our diet and they help in:

- Fighting heart disease, cancer, depression and hyperactivity

- Lowering bad cholesterol

- Increasing energy and the ability to concentrate

- Lowering the risk of getting a cold

- Transporting fat-soluble vitamins

- Satisfying hunger (keeping you full longer)

- Promoting weight loss

Unsaturated fats are divided into polyunsaturated and monounsaturated. It can sound confusing, so just remember that anything with the word 'unsaturated' in it is good fat. Both polyunsaturated and monounsaturated fats, if eaten in moderation and used to replace saturated or trans fats, can help lower your cholesterol levels and reduce your risk of heart disease.

Polyunsaturated fats: Found mostly in vegetable oils, these help lower both blood cholesterol and triglyceride levels. One type of polyunsaturated fat is omega-3 fatty acids with potential heart-health benefits that have received a lot of attention. Polyunsaturated fats provide us with essential fatty acids (EFA) like omega-3, which are essential for many biological processes from building healthy cells to maintaining brain and nerve function. To eat a variety of healthy fats and obtain adequate amounts of both fatty acids, include fish, nuts, seeds and vegetable oils. Increased EFA consumption has been found to lessen water retention and reduce the risk of kidney problems, celiac disease, cystic fibrosis, inflammatory bowel disease, cardiovascular disease, strokes and cancer.

Monounsaturated fats: These are heart-healthy fats and typically a good source of the antioxidant vitamin E, a nutrient often lacking in American diets. They can be found in:

- Olives
- Cashews
- Avocados
- Sesame seeds
- Hazelnuts
- Pumpkin seeds
- Almonds
- Olive oil
- Brazil nuts
- Peanut oils

BAD FATS: SATURATED (limit these!)

Saturated fats are found in animal products such as butter, cheese, whole milk, ice cream, cream and fatty meats. Although new studies show that there is no association between saturated fat and heart disease, for decades it has been believed that too much saturated fat can increase the amount of cholesterol in the blood, which increases the risk of heart disease and stroke.

HERE'S MY TAKE: Saturated fats are excellent cooking fats as they are highly resistant to heat-induced damage. For this reason, coconut oil and butter are fantastic choices for cooking, especially for high-heat cooking methods like stir-frying or frying. Additionally, 'healthy' saturated fats provide a concentrated source of energy in your diet, and give you the building blocks for cell membranes and a variety of hormones. Try to limit the intake of sat-fats to the most natural healthy version possible like coconut oil and butter.

WORST FATS: TRANS FAT AND HYDROGENATED OILS
(avoid completely!)

There are two types of fat you should try to avoid: trans fat and hydrogenated oils. Both can raise cholesterol levels, clog arteries and increase the risk of heart disease.

Trans fats are found naturally in very small amounts in meat and dairy products. Once again, natural trans fats are not the ones to be concerned about, especially if you choose low-fat dairy products and lean meats. The real worry in an American diet is the artificial trans fats that are used extensively in frying, baked goods, cookies, icings, crackers, packaged snack foods, microwave popcorn and some margarines. Also known as hydrogenated oils.

Much larger amounts are produced in the making of partially hydrogenated vegetable oils. Hydrogenation is a process that turns an unsaturated fat into a saturated fat and changes its molecular shape. When this happens, we're left with trans fats, which are, according to most experts, the most harmful fats of all. Trans fats produced in this way have been shown to have more adverse effects on blood cholesterol levels than saturates. They are difficult for our bodies to process and are commonly labeled as partially hydrogenated or just hydrogenated oils.

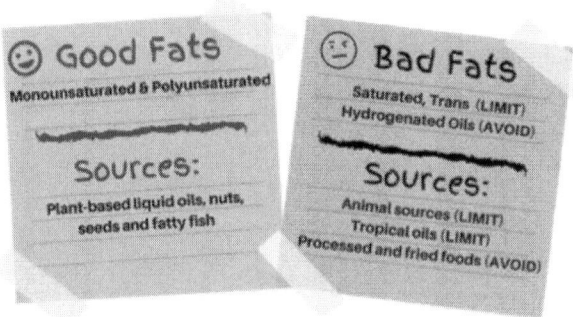

WANT TO GO NUTS?

Nuts and seeds are often seen as unwelcome because of their high calorie and fat content. But as you just learned, calories don't really matter, and there are good and bad fats. Nuts are packed with good fat, which is optimal for your health. These bite-size nutritional powerhouses, full of heart-healthy fats, protein, vitamins and minerals have a mix of omega-3 fatty acids that will help you in many ways. A number of studies have suggested that nuts can help cut the risk of heart disease[iii] and Type II diabetes, as well as aiding weight loss.

In one of the largest studies to date[iv], researchers from Harvard University have found that just a few servings of nuts per week may help keep your heart healthy. And more specifically, they found that walnuts and peanuts — but not peanut butter — may give your heart a boost.

Here are 10 reasons why you should try to incorporate them into your diet:

1. **Nuts can improve your digestion.** Rich in dietary fiber, nuts contribute to positive, normal function of your digestive system. A healthy gastrointestinal tract is key to a healthy body!

2. **They are high in fiber**, which will make you feel fuller, and reduce the risk of cancer and heart disease.

3. **They are a rich source of phytosterols and polyphenols.** Polyphenols are plant-derived antioxidants that protect the body from free radicals, so you can stay young and gorgeous. The phytosterols bind to cholesterol and help to sweep it out from your body. They are recognized by the American Heart Association as a natural way to reduce heart disease risk.

4. **Nuts contain healthy fats and oils.** Nuts are rich in the essential fatty acids linoleic acid and alpha linolenic acid: all great stuff for your health.

5. **They're a great source of B vitamins and vitamin E.** Nuts provide many vital B-complex vitamins such as riboflavin, niacin, thiamin, pantothenic acid, vitamin B6, and folate, which have tons of great benefits for your health.

6. **Nuts are the richest plant source of zinc and magnesium.** These are critical nutrients for immunity and reproductive function; a lot of people don't get enough of these at times.

7. **Nuts are portable and versatile.**

8. **They lower your weight.** Remember when we talked about fat and said that you need good fat to burn fat? Well, about one handful a couple of times a week should do the trick.

9. They support skin health. The make-up of most nuts includes zinc and vitamin E, both essential for smooth and healthy skin.

10. Nuts help stabilize your blood-sugar levels and improve your cholesterol.

The benefits of consuming nuts and seeds don't stop here. Some of my all-time faves are: almonds, pistachios, cashews, walnuts and peanuts. Try to integrate them into your diet and see how you feel. They are a great snack and could really help you with your cravings or mindless eating. But try to limit pecans and macadamia nuts as they have the lowest levels of proteins.

BEWARE! Just like with everything else, eating too much of a good thing does not make it great. The right portions of nuts should be as big as your palm (about six nuts) and you should not eat more than 20 nuts a day.

BOTTOM LINE: The type of fat you ingest becomes the type of fat you store in your body; so eating unnatural bad fats creates a pile of toxic fat residue in your body. Start reading labels and look for words like 'shortening', 'trans fat', and hydrogenated or partially hydrogenated oil. Remember, balance is key. Don't shy away from healthy fats as long as you're consuming them in moderate amounts. Fats break down fats, so it's necessary to include healthy fats in your diet to ensure that you are giving your body the tools it needs to break down and eliminate stored fat-soluble toxins.

OILS

Using proper oils is an important part of your detox. Some oils may help you reach your goals, while others may move you away from them. Oils are manufactured and extracted in different ways, and some ways are definitely less toxic to our bodies than others. Because of this, when shopping and cooking with oils, you will need to pick them carefully.

Here are a few criteria to help you choose and store them:

- **Stay away from refined oils** as they are highly processed with chemical compounds to extend their shelf lives. Always *read the labels* and look for keywords like 'unrefined', 'organic', 'expeller-pressed' or 'cold-pressed'; if the label does not list how the oil was extracted, it was most likely refined.

- **Choose oils that are bottled in dark or opaque glass**, as this will protect the oil from light and oxidation. Stay away from oils that are in clear or plastic bottles since inert gases are usually added to inhibit oxidation and the spoiling of the oil. The only oil you can buy in a clear glass container is coconut oil.

- **Store unopened bottles in a cool, dark place.**

- **Refrigerate oils after opening, except olive oil.**

- **Do not add new oil to a bottle of older oil.**

BEST OILS FOR COOKING:

- **Unrefined coconut oil:** Coconut oil is antibacterial, antiviral and antioxidant, great to cook at medium temperatures.

- **Avocado oil:** It has a light nutty flavor and can be used in stir-fries, for pan-frying or searing fish and meat.

- **Olive oil:** It should only be used to cook at low temperatures. It can add a great flavor to slow-roast vegetables in the oven.

BEST NON-COOKING OILS:

These oils are great raw, on salads, in smoothies and for popcorns or anything else you can imagine.

- Olive oil

- Flax oil

- Hemp oil

- Any other nut and seed oils like walnut, almond, and hemp.

OILS TO AVOID:

These oils contain trans fats, go rancid when exposed to oxygen and oftentimes are genetically modified. Personally, I choose to avoid these oils and use mainly extra-virgin olive oil and coconut oil.

- Canola oil: subject of much debate

- Cottonseed oil

- Partially hydrogenated oils

- Safflower oil

- Sunflower oil

- Vegetable oil

- Corn oil: usually GMO, processed and full of pesticides.

- Peanut oil: not available in organic varieties and some studies indicate that it may contain a toxic fungus contamination and contribute to atherosclerosis in some animals.

COCONUT OIL: THE TRUTH

For years, coconut oil has had a bad reputation because of its very high saturated fat content. Processed, refined tropical oils are dangerous. However, unrefined organic coconut oil has some distinct and powerful health benefits that should be promoted. Besides being ideal for occasional baking and cooking at low to medium temperatures, its stability stops the oil from creating free radicals, the molecules that wreak havoc on our cells.

Some proven benefits of coconut oil are:

- Lowering levels of cholesterol

- Preventing heart disease

- Preventing diabetes

- Killing bacteria, viruses and fungi, helping to stave off infections

- Stopping your hunger in its tracks, making you eat less without even trying; the fatty acids in coconut oil can significantly reduce appetite, which may positively affects body weight over the long term

- Helping to reduce seizures in epileptic children

- Protecting hair against damage, moisturizing skin and functioning as sunscreen

- Increasing your energy expenditure, helping you burn more fat

- Boosting brain function in Alzheimer's patients; studies show that the fatty acids in coconut oil can increase blood levels of ketone bodies, supplying energy for the brain cells of Alzheimer's patients and relieving symptoms

- Helping you lose fat

While research[v] shows coconut oil contains higher amounts of saturated fat and does increase total cholesterol (good and bad), those amounts do not increase your heart attack or stroke risk.

BOTTOM LINE: Everything in moderation. Just because something is good in small doses does not mean it's great if you have more. Don't make coconut oil your be all and end all, but add it to your diet here and there to experience some of the benefits.

A GRAIN OF TRUTH

Grains are small, hard, edible, dry seeds that grow on grass-like plants called cereals. Just like with carbs, whole grains can be divided into two categories: refined and unrefined (whole).

Whole grains: These contain all the essential parts and naturally occurring nutrients of the entire grain seed. Whole grains are as follows: amaranth, quinoa, millet, buckwheat, barley, bulgur, corn, einkorn, faro, kamut, millet, oats, rice, rye, sorghum, spelt, triticale, wheat and wild rice.

Refined grains: If the grain has been processed, it gets stripped of all its nutrients, leaving it empty of nutritional value and hard to digest, which will cause inflammation in your body. Refined grains include: white rice, white bread, regular white pasta, and other foods that have been made with white flour (also called 'enriched wheat flour' or 'all-purpose flour'), including many cookies, cakes, breakfast cereals, crackers and snack foods.

Although they have many health benefits, grains were not regularly consumed for most of human history. So, unless grains were a significant portion of your family dietary history, chances are that you might have a hard time digesting them, which could be toxic to your body. Grains contain toxic anti-nutrients, lectins, gluten and phytates, which are all not so great for you. For this reason, I believe that most people's health would benefit from avoiding all types of refined grains and some of the whole grains like:

CORN: Yes, corn is a grain not a vegetable! Besides the fact that nearly all corn and corn products in the American market contain GMO corn, corn and corn products are often difficult to digest and can contain mold toxins, which have been estimated to affect one in three people with allergies. Even small amounts of these fungal toxins can cause a range of health problems, including cancer, heart disease, asthma, multiple sclerosis and diabetes.

WHEAT, SPELT, BARLEY, KAMUT, TRITICALE and RYE:
These grains all contain gluten, a composite of the proteins gliadin and glutenin, which is harmful to your body. We will talk more in detail about gluten further on in the book. For now, just know it's not good news.

WHEAT: Most people believe that grains are a wholesome part of a healthy diet, particularly whole grains such as whole wheat. The truth is that eating wheat may not be beneficial to your health. Wheat is one of the most commonly used ingredients. Its hardy, glutinous consistency makes it practical for cakes, breads, pastas, cookies, bagels, pretzels and cereals. This ancient grain can actually be highly nutritious when grown and prepared in the appropriate manner. Unfortunately, our modern farming techniques and milling practices have dramatically reduced the quality of the commercial wheat berry and the flour it makes. Among many other issues, each grain of 'modern wheat' contains about one microgram of wheat germ agglutinin (WGA), which studies show may be pro-inflammatory, immunotoxic, cardiotoxic and neurotoxic. The result is that many people have become intolerant or even allergic to this nourishing grain[vi].

QUINOA: An important exception is quinoa, a vegetable seed that can have truly great health benefits for some people. Unfortunately, there are some who have problems digesting it, so if you consume it and find yourself always bloated, you might want to try to eliminate it from your diet.

All things considered, here are some of my favorite grains:

MILLET: Sweet and mild-tasting, it's high in magnesium, which has been shown to lower the risk of Type II diabetes.

Unfortunately, in the US, it is most commonly used only as birdseed.

OATS: Oats are the ultimate American breakfast staple and are just great! They are a complete source of protein, high in fiber with numerous health benefits including stabilizing blood sugar, lowering bad cholesterol and reducing blood pressure.

KEEP IN MIND: Oats are inherently gluten-free, but frequently contaminated with wheat during growing or processing, so if you are gluten-intolerant or celiac, always make sure to buy the gluten-free version.

BLACK, BROWN OR WILD RICE: These rice varieties have the highest amount of antioxidants of all rice, and even more than blueberries. These types of rice are also easily digested and rich in iron and fiber. (Another great option for digestion is basmati rice.)

Once again, like with everything in nutrition, it all depends entirely on your individual body's needs. If you like grains and feel good eating them, there's no good reason for you to avoid them as long as you're eating mostly *whole* grains. On the other hand, if you notice that eating grains makes you feel bad, then you might want to avoid them, because grains are not essential to your diet, and there is no nutrient in them that you can't get from other foods.

LEARN TO LISTEN TO YOUR BODY

Now that we have a clearer understanding of the basics of nutrition, it's time to learn how to listen to your body. We hear this all the time, but what does it really mean? And how do you do it? What if you feel like eating a cookie and sit in front of the TV instead of working out? What then? What kinds of feelings are you listening to when you do that?

Following your mind can certainly keep you busy. Indeed, at times, it can also be pretty overwhelming. So, how can you tell the difference between listening to your body instead of the voice inside your head? The answer is getting quiet and becoming sensitive to yourself. Your body is constantly sending you messages through gut feelings. All you need to do is turn those sensations into reason. Intellectualize them, if you like. Only then can you act on them.

Here are three easy steps to listen to your body:

1. Slow down! Think before you act. Don't jump in the kitchen the first signal you think you are getting. Instead, take a moment to pause and think.

2. Put your investigator hat on. Time to bring in some logic! Ask yourself, "What am I feeling?" and "Where is this thought coming from?"

Here's an example: If you are hungry, ask yourself, "Where is this thought coming from? Am I really hungry? Could I be thirsty? Am I simply bored or sad?"

If you are craving chocolate, you may be either lacking iron (for the ladies, this often happens before periods), or feeling sad or bored.

3. Act! Clarity equals power. Now that you are aware of the root of your thoughts, you can take action on them.

In the example above, instead of going for that instant gratification, and attacking the chocolate muffin or cookies, you can snack on an iron-rich product (spinach, apricot, raisins, etc.) or go for a jog to get the endorphins up to feel happy and clear your mind! See how this works?

CRAVINGS: THE TRUTH BEHIND THEM

Now, I know that cravings are real. I used to be obsessed with chocolate and sweets. I literally could not go a day without some. I am sure you may know exactly what I am talking about. Regardless of your cravings, have you ever craved carbs or something salty or fried? Yes? Well, here's the good news: Your body is not trying to sabotage you. It's not a weakness or 'just how it is'. Let me explain.

Your body is smart. When it is missing key nutrients or lacking emotional balance, it sends you signals like cravings. Any sort of imbalance in your nutrition or lifestyle can make your body ask you to 'fill the void'. Unfortunately, cravings always come when we least expect it and for those not-so-healthy foods.

You may feel hungry when you're actually thirsty. Again, cravings can strike because you are tired, stressed or unhappy. If you learn to decode these feelings, you can give your body exactly what is lacking, instead of jeopardizing all your efforts to live healthily and happily. Here's how to decode the four main cravings and a few alternative suggestions to deal with them:

CHOCOLATE: You may crave chocolate when your body is trying to compensate emotionally, for example, when you feel stressed or unhappy. Chocolate releases endorphins, those 'feel-good' hormones responsible for your feelings of happiness and comfort.

Cravings for chocolate could also indicate that your body is deficient in magnesium, which is actually a pretty common deficiency.

Add to your diet any of the following:

- Spinach
- Chard
- Pumpkin seeds
- Yogurt or kefir
- Almonds
- Black beans
- Avocados

- Figs
- Dark chocolate
- Banana
- Beets
- Onions
- Carrots
- Sweet potatoes

I truly do believe in the health benefits of cacao, so if you're going to eat chocolate, choose organic cacao and mix it into a healthy smoothie, or eat a small amount of organic dark chocolate with at least 80% cocoa.

SWEETS: Craving sweets can often be a sign of dehydration. Reach for some water and give your body 10 minutes to see if your sweet tooth goes away. Warm water with lemon is particularly helpful, as it helps flush out toxins faster.

Another reason for your sweet tooth could be that your body is trying to balance emotionally. In this case, try to find a way to treat or comfort yourself with something other than food. For me, having a massage, doing some yoga or taking a bubble bath works wonders.

Also, try incorporating more sweet fruits and veggies into your daily diet like:

- Sweet potatoes
- Beets
- Beans
- Butternut squash
- Onions
- Pumpkin
- Carrots
- Apples (a quick wonderful fix to help stave off the need for something sweet)

SALTY FOODS: A craving for salty food may signal a couple of things.

- **Lack of sodium in your diet:** We should include salt in our diets, but it is recommended to avoid plain old table salt. Try to switch to an unrefined mineral or sea salt. Himalayan and Celtic salts are my two favorites; they contain various minerals and provide the right amount of sodium for your body.

- **Lack of minerals in your body:** Incorporate pumpkin seeds, sunflower seeds, flax and dark chocolate to boost your intake of important minerals. Sea vegetables are a great source of minerals too. Powdered kelp is easy to throw into a smoothie and nori seaweed can be added to your water when boiling rice or pasta.

- **Your body is dehydrated:** Exercise, alcohol consumption and even a high salt diet can all lead to dehydration. Another good indicator is the color of your pee. If yellow and smelly, you are likely dehydrated.

Reach for some water, and if you can, go to your health food store and grab some water with electrolytes in it.

FATTY FOODS: Your craving for fatty, fried foods is usually your body's way of asking you to consume more fats. Remember though, not all fats are created equal! If you find yourself craving fries, fried chicken, cheese or anything oily, try to add to your diet healthier fats like: avocados, raw nuts (such as almonds and cashews), and coconut or olive oil.

I have created a complete list of possible cravings and what to eat to get rid of them. You can find it in the next page.

CRAVINGS

IF YOU CRAVE THIS	YOU ARE LACKING THIS	YOU SHOULD EAT MORE OF...
Chocolate or Acid Foods	Magnesium	Raw nuts and seeds, legumes, fruits, spinach, chard, pumpkin seeds, yogurt or Kefir, almonds, black Beans, avocado, figs, dark chocolate, banana, beets, onions, carrots, sweet potatoes
Sweet foods	Chromium Carbon Phosphorus Sulfur Tryptophan Emotional grounding	Broccoli, grapes, cheese, dried beans, calves liver, chicken, Fresh fruits, Chicken, beef, liver, poultry, fish, eggs, dairy, nuts, legumes, grains, cranberries, horseradish, cruciferous vegetables, kale, cabbage cheese, liver, lamb, raisins, sweet potato, spinach beets, onions, carrots, sweet potatoes, beans, squash
Salty Foods	Chloride	Raw goat milk, fish, unrefined sea salt
Cool Drinks	Manganese	Walnuts, almonds, pecans, pineapple, blueberries
Soda / Carbonated Drinks	Calcium	Mustard and turnip greens, broccoli, kale, legumes, cheese, sesame
Bread / Toast	Nitrogen	High protein foods: fish, meat, nuts, beans
Oily snacks / Fatty foods	Calcium Healthy fats	Mustard and turnip greens, broccoli, kale, legumes, cheese, sesame, avocado, nuts, coconut oil, olive oil
Coffee or Tea	Phosphorous Sulfur NaCl (salt) Iron	Chicken, beef, liver, poultry, fish, eggs, dairy, nuts, onion, legumes, egg yolks, red peppers, muscle protein, garlic, cruciferous vegetables, sea salt, apple cider vinegar Meat, fish and poultry, seaweed, greens, black cherries
Alcohol / Drugs	Protein Avenin Calcium Glutamine Potassium	Meat, poultry, seafood, dairy, nuts, granola, oatmeal, mustard and turnip greens, broccoli, kale, legumes, cheese, sesame, supplement glutamine powder for withdrawal, raw cabbage juice, sun-dried black olives, potato peel broth, seaweed, bitter greens
Tobacco	Silicon Tyrosine	Nuts, seeds; avoid refined starches, Vitamin C supplements or orange, green and red fruits and vegetables
Chewing ice	Iron	Meat, fish, poultry, seaweed, greens, black cherries
PRE-Menstrual cravings	Zinc	Red meats , seafood, leafy vegetables root vegetables
General overeating	Silicon Tryptophan Tyrosine	Nuts, seeds; avoid refined starches, cheese, liver, lamb, raisins, sweet potato, spinach, vitamin C supplements, orange, green, red fruits and vegetables

Whatever you do, the most important takeaway is to learn to trust your body. Distinguish physical food cravings from emotional cravings, listen to your body's clues, cater to its needs, and before you know it, you will be craving-free for good.

Want to try something fun? Learn to crave the good stuff. Research from Tufts University shows that we can rewire our brain circuits to prefer healthy foods! The trick is to choose those foods when you are extremely hungry. "Hunger helps form neurological connections between taste and pleasure," explains Susan B. Roberts, PhD and Tufts Professor of Nutrition and Science. By eating your snack 10 to 15 times on an empty stomach, Roberts says that you can fast-track the formation of a new habit. Some women in Roberts' weight loss groups say that they changed their cravings in just two weeks!

BEAT THE BINGE

Emotional eating is more common than you might think, as you don't always have to empty your fridge in the middle of the night to fall into this category. In fact, it's considered emotional eating when you find yourself eating for reasons other than satisfying actual physical hunger. This usually happens for four reasons:

1. If you skip meals or restrict your calories.

When you allow yourself to get overly hungry, it's nearly impossible to listen to your body, tune into hunger and fullness cues, or stop eating when you're satisfied. Check out the section on the truth about calorie-counting to stop this cycle.

2. If you deprive yourself of what you really want to eat.

When you hold yourself back from certain foods, you're depriving your body of what it's truly hungry for. To purposely end this cycle, think about addition instead of restriction. When you add something, something else naturally has to fall away. Check out the sections on calories and cravings to understand how to tune in to your body and break this pattern for good.

3. You eat mindlessly to avoid situations or a task.

Eating to keep yourself from doing what you should be doing rather than confronting the task or situation falls into the category of emotional eating. Since this is only a temporary fix, try instead to write on a piece of paper everything you are procrastinating on, then take out your calendar and schedule a specific time to do each of the tasks on your to-do list. This should give you an immediate sense of relief and peace, and will help you break the pattern.

4. You turn to food when strong emotions or uncomfortable feelings arise.

If you immediately turn to food after a stressful situation, to cover up sadness, soothe loneliness or fill emptiness, you are officially a victim of emotional eating. This will distract you from your emotions, but will not resolve the issue in the long run. You need to address the feelings and where they are coming from.

This topic touches me deeply as I was an emotional eater for quite some time. Here are a few more suggestions that helped me overcome this pattern:

1. Ditch cheat days.

Sometimes I used to claim an entire cheat day. I was 'good' during the week, then when Saturday or Sunday would roll around I would go crazy and eat anything I wanted for breakfast, lunch, dinner and snacks. The problem with this is that if you only allow yourself to enjoy 'forbidden' foods for one single day, you're more likely to overeat them on those occasions when you are 'allowed' them, even eating foods you don't care for because they're off limits every other day of the week. One bad *meal* will not undo your progress, but a whole day will. So as long as you follow the principles in this book, if one day a week you crave something in particular and you just want to treat yourself, go for your life and enjoy yourself! What I am asking you to try is to limit any indulgence to one or two meals a week, not a full day. Once you get past the next 11 weeks, then you will revisit this concept.

2. Eat only when you're actually hungry.

If you are an emotional eater, it's likely that you tend not to eat when you're hungry, which will only make you want to eat more later on. Listen to your body and feed it what it is asking for, when it is asking for it. Your body knows what it needs and when it needs it, so you learn to provide it with all the nutrition necessary for it to work properly. Always remember to be mindful about your choices, and whenever a craving arises refer back to the chart before to give your body with it actually needs.

3. Prepare for your next binge by knowing your triggers.

Discover your triggers and strategize. If you know you eat when you're lonely, plan to call a friend or write in your journal instead. Also, always carry food with you so that you never feel deprived. Stock your fridge with delicious, healthy foods, pack your calendar with exciting things to do, and be disciplined about setting aside time for yourself to relax.

4. Drink water.

Often times we confuse thirst with hunger. Next time you are hungry, reach for a glass of water and wait 10 minutes. Still hungry? Eat on, sista!

5. Start a food journal.

Journaling can be a powerful instrument to bring awareness to what you eat and to shine a light on the feelings connected to your need to eat. It has helped many of my clients in the past so you may find it useful too. There are many Apps available to track your food intake although I am not a fan as they track calories. Rather, I suggest you start a note on your phone to log daily what foods you are consuming but *most importantly how are you feeling* at the time of eating. Are you sad? Angry? Happy? Stressed? Ask yourself why are you feeling a certain way, write it down and review once a week. Logging your feelings at the time of eating will bring major insight to which areas of your life needs some adjustment.

6. Get support.

Sometimes, our emotions are so deeply rooted and we are so involved in how we're feeling that it's hard for us to understand the real reason behind our binging patterns. Find a mentor, a personal coach or a therapist to help you gain clarity on the real reason behind your binging habits to help you break through.

REMEMBER: Changing a behavior can feel overwhelming at first, so do what feels right for you, but keep in mind that it may get worse before it gets better. Keep going and you will find incredible happiness on the other side. You're not alone!

SUPPLEMENTS

Many people still question the importance of taking supplements, especially their benefits, effectiveness and even safety. Truth is that there's no general rule for how much of what supplement every person should take, or even if they should take any at all. Yet I truly believe in supplementing and strongly encourage you to explore this world.

Eating the right nutrients will make your body function properly, assisting your body during the detox process that it inevitably goes through as you clean up your lifestyle and allowing you to achieve optimal help faster. Especially with weight loss, nutrients play a critical role, as eating the adequate amount of vitamins and minerals will help you burn calories more efficiently, regulate appetite, lower inflammation, aid digestion, regulate stress hormones, and help your cells become more insulin-sensitive. It's important that you consult with your physician before starting any supplementation, as certain supplements require a blood test to ensure you have a need for that specific nutrient. For example, magnesium, iron, vitamin D.

But why do we need to supplement anyway? Especially in the past 100 years, methods of farming, manufacturing and cooking have changed drastically, causing foods to be stripped of important nutrients. In fact, current commercial agricultural techniques leave the soil deficient in important minerals, causing food to share the same mineral deficiencies. Additionally, shipping and storage techniques cause further depletion of vitamins, including the important B-complex and C vitamins. Erratic eating habits, insufficient chewing of food, eating on the run and stress also contribute to poor digestion and makes it harder for the body to extract all the nutrients it needs from food. This is why nutritional supplements can come in handy.

Here are a few supplements worth investigating:

1. Probiotics

The body is full of bacteria, both good and bad. Probiotics are the yeast and good bacteria that are essential to our health, especially our digestive system. We naturally have them in our bodies, but chronic use of antibiotics, medications, drinking tap water and stress are some of the factors that can contribute to lower levels of these good bacteria in our bodies. Probiotic supplements help rebalance your 'good' and 'bad' bacteria levels so your body can thrive. If you suffer with constipation, acne, bad mood, diarrhea, allergies, gas, IBS, IBD, bladder and/or yeast infections, you might want to look into these.

2. Spirulina

Spirulina is a spiral-shaped blue-green algae that grows in freshwater lakes and ponds around the world. Originally used as a complete source of protein by ancient Aztec and African populations, this nutrient-packed organism has a powerful blend of highly alkalizing, detoxifying and energy-boosting vitamins and minerals. Spirulina often comes in powdered form. Personally, I like to add it to my smoothies. Its distinct earthy flavor may not be for everyone, so just know that caps are also available to make it easier to integrate into your everyday lifestyle.

3. Fish oil

Omega-3s are powerful anti-inflammatories. I strongly believe fish oil is an essential supplement and highly recommend it to everyone, especially those not eating meat or fish. In fact, despite the fact that it's not vegan and there are many other sources of omega-3, the most beneficial essential fatty acids (EFAs) required for fighting and preventing physical and mental disease can only be found in fish or krill oil. EFAs are extremely important for brain health, and proper thyroid and adrenal activity.

Omega-3s will increase your energy levels, improve your ability to concentrate and help fight or prevent heart disease, cancer, depression, Alzheimer's, arthritis, diabetes, hyperactivity and many other diseases, even a simple flu. On the other hand, omega-3 deficiencies have been tied to:

- Mental fog (unable to think
- straight)
- Weight gain
- Depression
- Allergies
- Arthritis
- Brittle fingernails
- Dry skin and hair
- Chronic fatigue
- Lack of concentration
- Memory problems

It is normal to burp fishy for the first two weeks. If fish oil really won't cut it for you, flax oil is another option for EFAs, but keep in mind that is much harder for your body to convert to a usable form.

4. Digestive enzymes

I bet you've heard of digestive enzymes before and may have a vague idea of what they are, so let me clarify what I mean here. When we eat food, our digestive system absorbs its **nutrients**. Digestive enzymes are primarily produced in the pancreas and small intestine. These are responsible for breaking down food into nutrients so that your body can absorb them and use them to function properly. If you don't have enough digestive enzymes in your body, you cannot absorb all the nutrients in your food, so even though you may be eating healthily, you could be wasting all that good work.

You may not be aware of just how necessary enzymes are to every cell in your body — not just for digestion but for all your physiological processes. Insufficient enzyme production is at the root of much 'tummy trouble' in our country. Digestive problems cost Americans $50 billion each year, both in direct costs and absence from work. Chronic malabsorption can lead to a variety of illnesses. Think about it... If your body doesn't have the basic nutritional building blocks it needs, your health and ability to recover from illness will be compromised.

So, how do you know if you should you be taking them?

Some of the symptoms you might want to investigate with your doctor are:

- Low-grade inflammation in the digestive tract (food allergies, intestinal permeability, dysbiosis, parasitic infection, etc.)
- Low stomach acid
- Aging
- Chronic stress

- Gas and bloating after meals
- A sensation of food sitting in your stomach after you eat
- Feeling full after eating a few bites of food
- Undigested food in your stool
- Floating stools (an occasional floating piece is fine, but if all your poop consistently floats, that might be a sign something is wrong)
- An 'oil slick' in the toilet bowl (undigested fat)
- Constipation
- Bloating
- Cramping
- Flatulence and belching
- Heartburn and acid reflux

Digestive enzymes are very safe and reasonably cheap, so if you experience any of the above symptoms, you can give them a try and see if you notice any difference within a few weeks. The best way to determine if you specifically need them is through a stool exam, but keep in mind that most don't usually run this test and it's often not covered by insurance.

5. Vitamin D

Vitamin D is an extremely important vitamin that has powerful effects on several systems throughout your body. Vitamin D is necessary for strong bones, repair and maintaining steroid hormone that serves multiple gene-regulatory functions in your body. It's very important to have your vitamin D level checked, especially if you live in the northern part of the globe, where the sunlight is deficient.

Some signs of vitamin D deficiencies are:

- Getting sick or infected often
- Fatigue and tiredness
- Bone and back pain
- Depression
- Slow healing of wounds
- Hair loss
- Muscle pain

PLANNING AHEAD

"If you fail to plan, you are planning to fail."

Most people have a hard time implementing suggestions and changes in their lifestyle unless they sit down once a week, at a time when they are well-rested and relaxed, and plan for the week ahead. This is usually what I would do as a coach with my clients on our weekly check-in calls, but since this book is meant to hand you all the tools to help yourself, I will explain in detail how to do this.

The name of the game is 'think ahead'! The goal is to prevent yourself self-sabotaging all the efforts you have made to incorporate changes to your lifestyle. What we need to plan is: meals, social life, exercise and time for grocery shopping.

Here's how we are going to plan. Pick a day and time for the following:

Grocery shopping: Choose a specific day and time when you'll shop each week and write it in the planner. Keep a shopping list ready with you at all times. I love the app ShopShop. Since it's on my phone, I am always ready to add whatever I need whenever I think of something as the week goes on. This app also allows you to have different lists, scratch off the items you buy and keep items saved for future use. When you come home from grocery shopping, wash, cut up and store your veggies. This will extend the time that groceries take each week, but it will save you time cooking and cleaning afterwards.

Exercise: If you don't already, get in the habit of moving your body at least twice a week, ideally three times. For now, it doesn't matter what you do, as long as you move your body for a minimum of 30 minutes at least twice a week. It can be a walk in the park, taking your dog for a walk or whatever you like. Just make sure you don't skip it. To make this more likely to stick, identify the top three obstacles that could get in your way. For example, if you choose going for a walk outside or doing a workout outdoors, have a backup plan in case the weather is bad. For example, using the treadmill at a gym, working out at home, etc.

Social gatherings or dining out: Eating out is always hit or miss. Although we said that one bad meal will not undo your progress, if you eat out multiple times a week, it is a good idea to strategize to avoid coming home feeling guilty or worse. We have no control over what restaurants put in our food when we eat out, so if you eat out for lunch every day for work, try to plan ahead where and what you are going to eat so that you don't give in to temptation in the moment. If this sounds like you, I will give you some more ideas on how to protect your health bubble in social gatherings in Week 12 under the section on eating out.

Meals: I am not a particular fan of meal-planning, as it feels restrictive to me, but I do recognize it has helped many of my clients, especially busy moms and professionals. In order to plan meals strategically, it is a good idea to pick a few recipes you enjoy so you know exactly what you need to buy ahead of time. It has been estimated that most families consume only **10 to 15 recipes in their lifetime** and up to 30 in just a few cases. My suggestion? Pick your first 10 and try to keep it simple, so that all your meals are always quick and easy to prepare, and you don't waste a lot of time in the kitchen.

Before deciding what recipe you will cook and when, make sure to check your fridge and look for any food that is close to its expiration date. The recipes that use these ingredients will need to be assigned to the first days on your schedule. Make sure to take leftovers into account too.

Once all your meals and weekly routine is planned, stick the menu on the refrigerator so there is no question as to what you are doing or eating during the week. By deciding ahead of time what you will eat, it will allow you to go to the store when necessary or defrost the appropriate food from the freezer.

Since this section is all about planning everything, here are my last two suggestions.

First, surround yourself with **healthy snacks** (see snacks section at the back of the book). This will help you never make another unhealthy choice when you're hungry again! I keep my own secret stashes of healthy treats in my car, desk drawer and purse. Think of where you spend the most time... That's where you need to leave some nuts, carrot sticks or any of the other snack options you find at the end of this book.

And lastly, try to **avoid temptation**. Anything that triggers you to make an unhealthy choice needs to be eliminated — at least for now. For example, if every day you need to walk or drive past a bakery or somewhere that the irresistible aroma makes it impossible to stay away, walk or drive a different direction. Pretty simple, no?

ADD COLOR TO YOUR PLATE

What colors have you eaten today? You've probably heard this before. You need to eat the rainbow. But why is this suggestion so important? The focus here is on encouraging you to eat more whole fresh produce with a variety of fruit and vegetables, which have different colors. Eating 'more color in your food' will aid the detoxification process and ensure your body has many vitamins, minerals, antioxidants and phytonutrients that can't be replicated in a supplement. Dietary diversity has also been demonstrated to decrease the incidence of cardiovascular disease, cancer, obesity and all causes of health-related mortality.

Let's take a look at the detail of what each color has to offer:

Red: Tomatoes, watermelon, red apples, beets, cherries, cranberries, red pears, pomegranate, strawberries, raspberries, red peppers, radishes, red potatoes, radicchio, red onions and pink grapefruit.

Red fruits and veggies are loaded with lycopene, anthocyanins and resveratrol, which are:

- Powerful anticancer agents

- Protective against heart disease

- Good for improving the skin's ability to protect itself against damaging UV rays

- Helpful in maintaining a healthy prostate

Yellow, Orange: Apricots, cantaloupe, galia melon, mangoes, nectarines, peaches, papaya, oranges, satsumas, grapefruit, pineapple, passionfruit, carrots, swede, sweet potatoes, butternut squash, pumpkin, yellow and orange peppers, sweetcorn, guava, persimmons, kumquat.

Orange foods are full of carotenoids, vitamin A and C, which are great for:

- Reducing your risk of developing cancer

- Supporting a healthy immune system

- Promoting bone growth

- Helping to regulate cell growth and division

- Post-workout snacks since carotenoids help repair micro tears in worked muscles

- Healthy vision

- Potassium and vitamin C

Green: Avocados, green apples, green grapes, honeydew, kiwi, limes, green peas, artichokes, kale and any other leafy greens, asparagus, broccoli, cauliflower, Brussels sprouts, Chinese and green cabbage, celery, cucumbers, leeks, endives, green peppers, collard greens, bok-choy, green onions, snap peas, snow peas, lettuce, spinach, zucchini, watercress.

Although we have all been raised with the classic phrase "eat your greens," fewer than 10% of American actually eat the suggested amounts of veggies. Green foods are a powerhouse. In fact, they are a rich source of chlorophyll, lutein, sulforaphane and indoles, and contain loads of B vitamins, which are all great for:

- Keeping your vision sharp and clear

- Boosting immunity

- Pumping up the detox system

- Boosting metabolism

- Lowering your blood sugar

- Reducing blood pressure

- Fighting cancer

- Fighting inflammation

- Cutting cholesterol

- Fiber

Blue, Purple, Crimson, Brown: Berries, cherries, plum, purple grapes, red wine, dark chocolate, cocoa, purple figs, purple cauliflower, purple carrots, purple cabbage, purple Belgian endive, raisins, concord grapes, forbidden (black) rice, acai, eggplant, purple potatoes, blackcurrants, blackberries, elderberries, purple kale, purple asparagus and purple artichoke.

Blue, purple, crimson, even brown foods are gaining popularity due to the fact they contain flavonoids, powerful antioxidants beneficial to our health because they contribute to:

- Maintaining proper brain function

- The maintenance of proper blood flow and blood vessels

- Fighting ulcers

- Keeping your liver healthy

- Lowering bad cholesterol

- Preventing UTIs

- Suppressing tumor growth

- Protecting against cancer

White, Tan, Brown: Bananas, cauliflowers, dates, white nectarines, brown pears, garlic, onions, ginger, mushrooms, potatoes, turnips, shallots, white corn.

Tan is not usually the most exciting color on the spectrum, but tan-colored foods still come packed with many health benefits. In fact, they can:

- Potentially reduce the risk of coronary heart disease

- Maintain a healthy digestive tract

- Reduce the risk of some types of cancer

- Add fiber to your diet

- Have powerful detoxifying sulfur compound

- Fight inflammation

- Contain cancer-fighting properties

- Be a good source of vitamin C and potassium

- Potentially ward off stomach and colon cancers

- Be packed with vitamin D, calcium and phosphorus, which aid in bone health and may help us maintain a healthy body weight

Just by remembering to eat a rainbow, you can increase your intake of nutrients and healthful food components. So, the next time you reach for one of the abovementioned foods, know that it is not only bursting with color and flavor, but also contains a component that may improve your health.

Now you know the different roles in the body, aim for at least three colors of food at every meal so that you can meet the recommended three servings of vegetables over the course of the day.

TRY: GET INTO YOUR NEW RHYTHM

This week we have covered a lot of topics. We first dove into some basics of nutrition to lay the foundation for a healthier future.

The most powerful step you can take to detox your body and restore it to wellness is creating a routine. Your body has a biological clock, which is a perfect machine that records everything. Whether you like it or not, or listen to it or not, it is subject to very specific rhythms. By scheduling specific times for your meals, sleep, workouts and relaxation, your body will be able to shift focus and energy to heal itself. Only then will the extra weight come off and stay off for good.

Simple lifestyle changes to help your body rebalance your daily rhythms can have surprisingly powerful effects:

increased energy, better sleep, weight loss, and much more. This is why I encourage you to set a daily schedule of sleeping, eating, exercising and relaxing for the next 11 weeks to help your body self-regulate into health and natural weight loss.

Here are a few tips for you to consider when planning your new schedule.

START YOUR MORNING RITUAL: In the next 11 weeks, it would be great for you to start your morning with your choice of: a cap of apple cider vinegar + juice of ½ small lemon, or a glass of warm (not hot) water + juice of ½ small lemon, or a glass of warm water + unsweetened aloe juice. Personally, I like to alternate them. By doing so, you will aid your body's natural detox process, helping it flush toxins, boost metabolism, stabilize blood-sugar levels, control cravings and aid digestion. Lots of benefits for such a simple routine, right?

DO NOT SKIP BREAKFAST: Whether you think that skipping breakfast will reduce your overall calorie intake for the day, you 'have no time' or are not hungry in the morning, you need to understand that this habit can be the cause of weight gain and low energy issues. By not eating a morning meal, you will actually eat *more* throughout the day. Eating a healthy breakfast will jumpstart your metabolism, help you burn more energy, and control your appetite and cravings. Studies repeatedly show daily breakfast consumption is associated with maintaining a healthy weight. If you're not ready for breakfast when you first wake up, listen to your body. Try getting a smoothie, a protein shake or eat whenever you feel ready, but do not skip it completely. If you don't have time to prepare breakfast in the morning, make it at night and grab it to go before heading out the door.

SLOW DOWN YOUR EATING: Do you know that it takes 20 minutes for the body's hunger signals to shut down after you start eating? Eat slowly, stop when you feel 80% full and wait before going back for seconds.

EAT MORE FREQUENTLY: It's important to balance your food intake throughout the day to help maintain normal blood sugar and decrease the chances of binging when hunger strikes. Feeding your body on a regular basis (every three hours) will keep your metabolism working, letting your body know that food is available and it's okay to burn energy rather than conserve and store it as fat. Be mindful on your snack choices. Check out the article on the blog section of my website www.eleonoracbastos.com for the best healthy snacks.

AVOID EATING FOOD TWO TO THREE HOURS BEFORE GOING TO BED: This will allow you to burn the food you consume for energy and help the body restore while you are sleeping. Whether you like it or not, at night, your body is in repair, rebuild, and growth mode, but the last thing you want to see grow is your belly. That's why observing this eating rule is important.

SLEEP SEVEN TO EIGHT HOURS: Research suggests that those who sleep five hours or less weigh five pounds more than those getting at least seven hours of shut-eye per night. Lack of sleep disrupts circadian rhythms and can lead to inefficient body regulation of energy balance, metabolism and appetite. Leptin and ghrelin levels — hormones that tell your body you're full and to stop eating – can become imbalanced with too little sleep. Said simply: Sleep more, eat well, and weigh less! Strive for seven to eight hours of sleep each night.

DRINK AT LEAST EIGHT GLASSES OF FILTERED WATER THROUGHOUT THE DAY. Did you know that hunger is often confused with dehydration? Next time you feel like having a snack, have a glass of water instead. Your pee is a good measure of your hydration too: It should be a pale yellow, if not completely clear, to be healthy! Even mild dehydration can alter your body's metabolism.

Ideally, you should aim to drink half of your weight (as a number, in pounds) in ounces of clean, filtered water. Also limit soda, caffeine, and alcohol as they all dehydrate you. If you are not a 'big drinker', try to start with eight glasses a day.

> **A LITTLE TRICK:** Set your alarm to go off every hour from the time you wake up. For the next eight hours, drink a full glass of water every time the alarm goes off. If you are at work, even better! Use the water as a five-minute break to restore your mind and unwind as well. Studies also show that those who drink one to two glasses of water before meals feel fuller and tend not to overeat so much.

THROW THE SCALE OUT THE WINDOW. Stressing out over your weight actually does more harm than good (we'll dive in deeply into this topic on chapter 10). The scale is an oversimplified, misleading manipulator that has wielded too much power over your life for too long and it's now time to end this unhealthy relationship. The problem with the scale is that we trust that number so much that it blinds us from success and can lead us down a trail of endless frustration. If your weight is going up you feel bad and if your weight is going down you feel good. Well, the truth is that the number on the scale doesn't differentiate between fat and muscle weight.

Therefore, you could be working out and eating well, but the number on the scale won't change.

If you bought this book is likely that your relationship with your weight isn't healthy. So since you are more likely to stress, obsess, and be confused by the number on the scale, it's time to take a stand and change your relationship with the scale by throwing it out the window and focusing only on how you feel rather than paying attention at that silly number. Results from now on will be measured on how your clothes fit but more importantly on how you feel, your energy levels and how often you're laughing and smiling.

I personally have not weighted myself in 5 years and I am still wearing the same clothes! This trick is one that I love using with my clients and I cannot tell you how many of them have thanked me for this!

BOTTOM LINE: The first step to take charge of your health is to make sure you understand the basics of nutrition. Once that is clear, you need to learn to give your body with the nutrients it needs to function properly. Science shows that skipping meals, eating very late, stressing over your weight and not having breakfast are all guaranteed ways to screw up your metabolism and gain weight. So, by all means, attack your health goal, but do it right so you set yourself up for lasting success!

CHECK-IN QUESTIONS

How were your energy levels on a scale of 1 to 10?

Did you feel fatigued or sluggish?

Can you think clearly?

Did you feel tired?

Did you feel bloated?

Did you have headaches? (If yes, how many?)

Did you go to the bathroom regularly?

Is your skin clear?

Did you have cravings?

Did you binge?

Did you eat or snack compulsively or mindlessly?

Is your sleep regular?

Did you have trouble concentrating or brain fog?

Did you suffer with mood swings?

Did you ever feel anxious, fearful, or nervous?

Did you feel physically weak?

Did you get sick?

Did you have bad breath?

Did you have heartburn?

Did you have stomach or intestinal pain?

Did you experience ringing in your ears?

Did you feel the need to urinate urgently or frequently?

Did you have pain or aches in your muscles and joints?

Did you feel stiff or limited in your movements?

"Nutrition labels should include a 'what if I ate the whole thing' section."

WEEK 3

THE KEY TO RAPID, NATURAL, LASTING WEIGHT LOSS

PROCESSED FOODS

This week, we are going to unveil the biggest labeling scams and learn how to outsmart clever marketing techniques. But before we do that, let's talk briefly about our bodies and why it matters to pay attention to what's in our food.

Processed, packaged foods have almost completely taken over the diet of Americans. It has been estimated that about 90% of the money that Americans spend on food is used to buy processed items. The reason behind this craze is probably the convenience factor. I get it. It's so much easier to cook rice for five minutes rather than 20, or bake a cake by pouring out a dry mix in a bowl, and adding an egg and some milk, rather than starting from scratch. But convenience isn't the only thing you get when you eat processed foods.

If you look at the ingredients labels on processed, packaged foods, chances are you won't have a clue what some of the ingredients are. That's because many of the ingredients in there aren't actual food… They are artificial chemicals that are added for various purposes. The most common ones are:

- Colorants
- Stabilizers
- Emulsifiers
- Bleach
- Texturizers

- Softeners
- Preservatives
- Sweeteners
- Odor-hiding agents
- Flavors

Besides the trouble caused by what's added to your food, there are a lot of essential components that are taken away. In fact, processed foods are often stripped of nutrients designed by nature to help digest and protect your health, such as soluble fiber, antioxidants, good fats and much more.

WHAT'S CONSIDERED A 'PROCESSED' FOOD ANYWAY?

There is big debate around this question, as processed foods can range from naturally preserved foods to completely denatured foods. Obviously, most of the foods we eat are processed in some way: apples are cut from trees, ground beef goes through a grinding machine and butter is cream that has been separated from the milk and churned. Also, there are foods that undergo minimal processing and remain highly nutritious, such as extra virgin olive oil, virgin coconut oil, raw apple cider vinegar, etc.

But there is a *huge difference* between *mechanical processing* and *chemical processing*. As a general rule of thumb, if it's a single-ingredient food with no added chemicals, then it doesn't matter if it's been ground or put into a jar. It's still real food. However, if it's boxed, bagged, canned or jarred, and has a list of five or more ingredients on the label, it's considered highly processed and therefore harmful to your health. Methods used to process foods include:

- Canning
- Freezing
- Refrigeration
- Dehydration
- Aseptic processing

Here's a shortlist of the most common processed foods that you should try to avoid:

- White wheat flour (or anything white, like bread, etc.)
- Refined sugars
- Margarine
- Refined vegetable oils (canola or rapeseed oil, soybean oil, canola oil, corn oil, sunflower oil, safflower oil, and peanut oil)
- Artificial sweeteners
- Food additives
- Canned foods
- Boxed foods (cereal, pasta, meal mixes, etc.)
- Soft drinks
- Sugary fruit drinks
- Fast food
- Cheese
- Packaged cookies, chips, cakes, snack foods, crackers, etc.
- Processed meat products (if they have artificial colors and soy filter)
- Frozen meals (fish sticks, pizza rolls and similar)

- Soy products (such as soy cheese, soy protein isolate)
- Powdered milk and eggs

WHAT IS WRONG WITH PROCESSED FOOD?

Now that you have a clearer idea on what processed foods are, here's why it's a good idea to eliminate them from your diet.

1. Processed food makes you fat

These foods are a product of chemical and mechanical manipulation. Many of them contain residues of pesticides, GMOs and synthetic chemicals that your body was never designed to ingest. When your liver does not know how to process these ingredients, it stores them as fat, oftentimes encapsulating them, creating those stubborn pockets of fat (love handle, culottes de cheval, etc.) that are almost impossible to lose.

2. Processed food impacts your mood

An interesting new study from the University of California, San Diego School of Medicine studied the diets and behaviors of nearly 1,000 men and women and found that a higher intake of trans fat was significantly tied to an increase in aggression and irritability. Previous studies have also linked trans fat to heart disease, infertility, cancer, Type II diabetes, liver problems and obesity, so avoiding it is a good move for your health and your mood.

According to the findings of another study published in 2014 conducted on 3,663 people, and published in the online *Public Library of Science* (PLoS) journal, long-term exposure to a diet high in processed foods and sugars is also a risk factor for depression.

3. Processed foods create cravings and addictions

The brain has a reward center, which lights up and starts secreting dopamine and other feel-good chemicals when we eat, which is why most of us 'enjoy' eating. Now, the funny thing is that our appetite gravitates towards foods that are sweet, salty and fatty, because we know such foods contain energy and nutrients that we need for survival. For this reason, food manufacturers 'got smart' and started spending massive amounts of money in research to find out how to make their foods as 'rewarding' as possible to the brain. As a result, processed foods, especially those high in added sugar and/or fat, release a much more powerful amount of feel-good chemicals compared to unprocessed foods (especially dopamine), which not only leads to over-consumption but creates addiction.

4. Junk foods cause inflammation, a leading factor in chronic illness

Studies show that refined sugars, processed flours, vegetable oils and other artificial ingredients are responsible for this plague. The next time you're craving candy or a bag of potato chips, think about how it's increasing your chances of heart disease, dementia, neurological problems, respiratory failure and cancer.

5. Processed foods are full of GMOs

The foundation of most processed foods in grocery stores today springs from laboratories, not nature. Genetically modified organisms (GMOs) have been linked to infertility, organ damage and cancer. Excessive amounts of these foods prompt weight gain, pollute your bloodstream, and can permanently affect the composition and function of your liver.

Keep in mind that processed foods can contain dozens of **additional chemicals** that aren't even listed on the label. For example, 'artificial flavor' is a proprietary blend. Manufacturers don't have to disclose exactly what that means and it can contain anywhere between 50 and 100 ingredients!

REDUCING PROCESSED FOODS: THE WHY

Given the prevalence of these nasty chemicals in processed foods, let's look at why you might think about reducing them.

Your liver has the most important job in your body's elimination process. When your body encounters toxins (chemicals), it has only a few ways to handle them: It encapsulates them as fat (those stubborn fat deposits that are almost impossible to eliminate), dumps them into tissue (such as muscle, organs and bone), or eliminates them through waste. If you think that, today, there are more than 3,000 chemicals added to food that the liver was never designed to handle, you can easily understand how your liver ends up overworked, stressed and burned out. An overloaded body will alert you that it is in a toxic state by sending out messages like:

- Fatigue

- Brain fog

- Headaches

- Chronic joint or muscle pain

- Digestion issues, including: gas, heartburn, bloating, diarrhea or constipation, and abdominal pain when eating

- Insomnia
- Autoimmune diseases
- Hormonal imbalances, like PMS or menopausal symptoms
- Acne or skin rashes
- Attention problems
- Anxiety or depression
- Allergies
- Inflammation
- Chemical sensitivities
- Chronic bad breath
- Weight gain

If you suffer from any of the above, don't worry, because you are not alone. The good news is that you can stop these symptoms by taking an active role in assisting your body to detoxify! How? The first step is to learn the most harmful chemicals and what they do to your health, so you can eliminate them ASAP.

THE MOST HARMFUL CHEMICALS

The list of common additives below does not include every single harmful additive out there, so arm yourself with a Google search when you see an ingredient that you are not familiar with or can't pronounce to make sure it's not dangerous to your health. The most common chemicals you have to watch out for are:

Butylated hydroxytoluene (BHT)

Found in: Processed foods, cosmetics, jet fuels, rubber petroleum products, transformer oil and embalming fluid.

Butylated hydroxyanisole (BHA)

Found in: Processed foods, especially in butter, beer, meats, cereals, chewing gum and many snack foods.

Both used as: Preservative. People also use it as medicine against genital herpes and HIV.

What they do to your body:

The International Agency for Research on Cancer classifies BHA as a possible *human carcinogen*. Long-term exposure to high doses of BHT is toxic in mice and rats, causing liver, thyroid and kidney problems and affecting lung function and blood coagulation[vii]. BHT can act as a tumor promoter in certain situations[viii].

High-fructose corn syrup (HFCS)

Used as: Sweetener.

Found in: Sodas, fruit-flavored drinks, cereal and most processed foods.

What it does to your body:

- Obesity

- Diabetes

- Metabolic syndrome

- High triglyceride levels

All these conditions boost your risk of heart disease. Time to rethink those 'strong heart antioxidants' cereal recipes!

Also, 90% of the time, HFCS is made from genetically modified corn and processed with genetically modified enzymes, which is a growing concern because they may have an unexpected and negative impact on human health, of which there is mounting scientific evidence.

To make matters worse, studies have recently revealed that nearly half of tested samples of HFCS contained mercury.

Soybean oil

Used as: Cheap vegetable oils for processed products AKA trans fat.

Found in: Commonly used to make mayonnaise, salad dressing, margarine, chocolate bars and non-dairy coffee creamers.

What it does to your body:

- Cancer, by interfering with enzymes your body uses to fight cancer

- Chronic health problems such as obesity, asthma, autoimmune disease, cancer, and bone degeneration

- Diabetes, by interfering with the insulin receptors in your cell membranes

- Decreased immune function, by reducing your immune response

- Reproductive problems, by interfering with enzymes needed to produce sex hormones

- Heart disease, by clogging your arteries

- Increased blood levels of low density lipoprotein (LDL), or 'bad' cholesterol, while lowering levels of high density lipoprotein (HDL), or 'good' cholesterol

- Interference with your body's use of beneficial omega-3 fats

Beyond the problems with soybean oil being a trans fat, two more concerns are the health hazards of the processed soy itself, as well as the prevalence of genetically engineered soybeans today.

Propylene glycol alginate (E405)

Used as: Emulsifier, stabilizer and thickener in food products. Even though propylene glycol is used as a food additive, it has many industrial uses including automotive antifreezes and airport runway de-icers.

Found in: Margarine, cake mixer, soda, pop and almost all carbonated drinks, frozen dessert and some ice creams, dressings, icing on cakes, chemical coffee (flavored coffee like nutmeg, vanilla, etc.), most types of gel-like foods, including yogurt, jellies and jams, ice cream and salad dressing. Certain condiments and chewing gum also contain it, as do some kinds of cosmetics.

What it does to your body:

- Irritation

- Nausea

- Coughing

- Wheezing

When it is used cosmetically, it can cause allergic reactions that include hair loss, rashes, and eye irritations.

Polysorbate 60 (polyoxyethylene-(20) sorbitan monostearate)

Used as: Made of corn, palm oil and petroleum. Used as replacement for dairy.

Found in: Cake mix, frozen dessert, salad dressing, donuts, foods with artificial chocolate coating, non-dairy whipped topping.

What it does to your body:

Although the FDA designated the chemical as 'safe for limited use', according to the *Journal of the National Cancer Institute*, the *Journal of Nutrition* and the *FAO Nutrition Meetings Report Series*, polysorbate 60 can cause:

- Detrimental reproductive effects

- Organ toxicity

- Cancer, if consumed in high doses

Monosodium glutamate (MSG)

Used as: Flavor enhancer.

Found in: Commonly added to Chinese food, canned vegetables, soups and processed meats.

What it does to your body:

Over the years, the FDA has received many anecdotal reports of adverse reactions to foods containing MSG, including:

- Spikes in insulin leading to uncontrollable hunger, cravings and overeating

- Headache

- Flushing

- Sweating

- Facial pressure or tightness

- Skin rashes

- Seizure

- Numbness, tingling or burning in the face, neck and other areas

- Rapid, fluttering heartbeats (heart palpitations)

- Chest pain

- Nausea

- Weakness

MSG, like most of these chemicals, has been used as a food additive for decades. The Food and Drug Administration (FDA) has classified MSG as a food ingredient that's 'generally recognized as safe', but its use remains controversial. For this reason, when MSG is added to food, the FDA requires that it be listed on the label. Please be aware that *textured soy protein concentrate, carrageenan, maltodextrin, disodium inosinate, disodium guanylate and modified cornstarch* are basically different names to hide ingredients that contain monosodium glutamate or form MSG during processing.

Diacetyl

Used as: Buttery flavor and aroma.
Found in: Microwave popcorn, fake butters, snack foods, pet foods, candies, baked goods and other food products.
What it does to your body: it has been linked to:

- Cancer

- Lung dysfunction

- Alzheimer

Several manufacturers have voluntarily removed the chemical from their products and some governments have stepped in to regulate the harmful chemical.

3-MCPD

Formed by: Exposing foods that contain fat and salt to high temperatures during the production process.

Found in: Asian oyster, soy and hoisin sauces. They're also found in wheat products, meat and cheese.
What it does to your body: it has been linked to:

- Cancer

- Genetic dysfunctions

- Male anti-fertility

Banned in the United Kingdom, Australia and New Zealand, though not yet in the United States, 3-MCPD is toxic to humans and raises your risk of cancer.

Palm oil, shortening, corn oil

Also known as: Partially hydrogenated oil trans fat.

Found in: Palm oil is the most widely consumed vegetable oil on the planet. These oils are in about half of all packaged products sold in the supermarket.

What it does to your body:

- Raised cholesterol

- Increased risk of heart attack

- Increased risk of blood clots

- Hypertension (elevated blood pressure)

- Clog your arteries

- Obesity

- Risk of metabolic syndrome

When a regular fat like corn, soybean or palm oil is blasted with hydrogen and turned into a solid, it becomes a trans fat. Choose healthier monounsaturated fats, such as olive, peanut and coconut oils, and foods that contain unsaturated omega-3 fatty acids instead.

Enriched flour and white processed foods

Found in: Foods that are white in color, like pasta, rice, bread, cake, cookies, brownies, pretzels, donuts, pie-crust, crackers, pizza dough, you name it.

What it does to your body:

- Type II diabetes

- Obesity

To reach the white color, ingredients (flour, grains, etc.) are chemically bleached and stripped of their properties. Your body breaks them down too quickly, flooding the bloodstream with too much sugar at once. These quick highs and lows in your blood-sugar level are what can lead to the two causes listed above. The 'enrichment' of flour is made using toxic ingredients and a type of iron that is metallic, which your body cannot absorb. Replace processed grains with whole grains, like brown or wild rice, whole-wheat breads and pastas, barley and oatmeal.

Corn syrup

Used as: Used in foods to soften texture, add volume, prevent crystallization of sugar and enhance flavor.

Found in: Processed and mass-produced foods, candies, soft drinks and fruit drinks.

What it does to your body:
- Increases triglycerides
- Boosts fat-storing hormones
- Drives people to overeat and gain weight

Adopt my zero-tolerance policy and steer clear of this 'sweet poison'.

Artificial sweeteners

Also known as: Aspartame, Equal, NutraSweet, Sucralose, Splenda, acesulfame potassium, Ace-K, neotame, saccharin, Sweet'N Low.

Used as: Sugar substitute.

Found in: Any pre-packaged foods, not only sweet. (More on this in the chapter on sugar.)

What it does to your body:

- Obesity

- Metabolic syndrome

- Type II diabetes

- Hypertension and cardiovascular disease

Studies suggest that artificial sweeteners trick the brain, making people more likely to keep eating sweet treats with abandon, and affect *metabolism* and *insulin levels* changing the body's insulin response.

Sodium benzoate and potassium benzoate

Also known as: E211, E212

Used as: Preservative to prevent mold, bacteria and fungus from growing.

Found in: Most widely used in acidic foods such as salad dressings, jams and fruit juices, carbonated drinks and condiments.

What it does to your body:
- Cancer (when mixed with ascorbic acid (vitamin C), sodium benzoate transforms into benzene, a known carcinogen that also damages DNA)

- Thyroid issues/damage

Some studies have shown that sodium benzoate along with artificial food colorings can cause children with ADHD to be more hyperactive.

Dangerous levels of benzene can build up when plastic bottles of soda are exposed to heat or when the preservatives are combined with ascorbic acid. Be careful!

Butyrate hydroxyanisole (BHA)

Used as: Preservative for all oil-containing processed foods. Its job is to help prevent spoilage and food poisoning, but it's a major endocrine disruptor and can seriously mess with your hormones.

Found in: Packaged foods and cosmetics.

What it does to your body: Although it is GRAS (generally recognized as safe) by the FDA, it's been shown to *cause cancer in animals*, raising concerns among the healthy living community that the additive could be carcinogenic to humans as well.

Sodium nitrates and sodium nitrites

Used as: Two different preservatives.

Found in: Processed meats like bacon, lunchmeat, and hot dogs.

What they do to your body:

- Colon cancer

- Metabolic syndrome, which can lead to diabetes

Protect your health by always choosing fresh, organic meats.

Allura Red AC

Also known as: Red 40

Used as: A food dye manufactured from petroleum.
Found in: Anything red — sodas, cough syrup, candy, cereal bars, etc.

What it does to your body: it has been linked to:

- Attention deficit hyperactivity disorder (ADHD)

- Other hyperactive disorders

- Increased risk of cancer

For this reason, Allura Red AC is banned or discouraged in several parts of Europe.

Tartrazine

Also known as: Yellow #5.

Used as: Synthetic food dye.

Found in: Anything colored yellow — sodas, cereals, candies, ice cream, pickles, cookies, pre-packed macaroni and cheese, and more.

What it does to your body: it has been linked to:

- Behavioral issues

- Cancer

- Damaged organs

It's banned in some areas of Europe, but legal (and regulated) in the United States and Canada. Almost all colorants approved for use in food are derived from coal tar and may contain up to 10ppm of lead and arsenic. Also, and not surprisingly, most coal tar colors could cause cancer.

Blue, Green, Red, and Yellow

Used as: Food dye.

Found in: Anything colored that is not a whole food from cereals to drinks. The artificial colors blue 1 and 2, green 3, red 3, and yellow 6 are all in the same boat.

What they do to your body: Besides the previously linked symptoms, these colors have also been linked to:

- Thyroid cancer

- Adrenal cancer

- Bladder cancer

- Kidney cancer

- Brain cancers

Always seek out foods with *no artificial colors*, especially when shopping for your kids. Look for color-free medications and natural food products that don't contain artificial colors like these.

Carrageenan

Found in: Most infant formulas, most store-bought milk alternatives, many creams, creamers and dairy products, yogurt, chocolate, soymilk and ice cream. The ingredient even crops up in certain frozen dinners, soups and commercial broth products.

Used as: Anticaking agent. It is widely used in the food industry for its gelling, thickening and stabilizing properties. Derived from red seaweed, it's often added to beverages to keep the ingredients from separating.

What it does to your body: The research is shaky on carrageenan being a carcinogen or not. Animal studies have repeatedly shown that food-grade carrageenan causes gastrointestinal inflammation and higher rates of intestinal lesions, ulcerations, and even malignant tumors. However, there are no conclusive studies as at late 2018. I suggest playing it safe and avoiding carrageenan whenever possible. If the USDA does finalize the vote to prohibit carrageenan in its products, it will make things a lot easier.

Potassium bromate

Found in: Flour and baking goods.

Used as: Typically used as a flour improver (e number E924), it acts to strengthen the dough and allow higher rising.

What it does to your body: Although banned for use in foods by many countries (Europe, Canada, Brazil and more), in the USA, potassium bromate is typically used as a flour improver in baked goods. Potassium bromate is a carcinogenic toxin and competes with iodine in the body, especially when any iodine deficiency is present. It is also linked to kidney and thyroid tumors in test animals.

Castoreum

Also known as: Extract from the perianal (butt) glands of beavers. Ewww!

Found in: 'Natural flavor' ingredient in processed foods.

PLEASE NOTE: Added flavoring, both natural and artificial, could contain anywhere from 50 to 100 ingredients. And often, all of the extra ingredients in flavors aren't as innocent as you would hope. Try to steer clear of them.

Ammonium sulfate

Used as: Fertilizer. It's a salt compound to regulate acidity.

Found in: Some bread and flour products.

What it does to your body: Although it isn't toxic unless consumed in large quantities, this substance can cause:

- Irritation in the gastrointestinal tract

- Nausea

- Vomiting

- Diarrhea

ORGANIC vs GMO

Now that you have had a look at what the most common chemicals do to your body, it's time to talk about organic food.

First, what does organic actually mean? Organic simply refers to food **grown in nature**, as our great grandparents knew it. Basically, organic produce and organic ingredients are grown without the use of pesticides, synthetic fertilizers, sewage sludge, genetically modified organisms or ionizing radiation. When organic refers to animal produce (meat, poultry, eggs and dairy products), it means the animals were not given any antibiotics or growth hormones either.

And GMOs? These are organisms whose genes have been manipulated in a laboratory through genetic engineering (GE) to become resistant to new pesticides and chemicals used in today's conventional farming methods. Are they safe? Most developed nations **do not consider GMOs to be safe**. In more than 60 countries around the world, including Australia, Japan and all countries in the European Union, there are significant restrictions or bans on the production and sale of GMOs. Unfortunately, in the US, the studies on the safety of GMOs have been conducted by the same corporations that created them and profit from their sale, and the government approved their use.

HERE'S THE TRUTH: Modern conventional farming methods that involve the use of GMOs and all other chemicals do not exist until the last century, which means that our bodies and genes weren't made to recognize them, process them and expel them properly.

Now, it is not possible to prove a food is safe, only to say that no hazard has been shown to exist. Establishing long-term safety would require prohibitively expensive decades of study of hundreds of thousands of GMO consumers and their non-

GMO counterparts. That will take time. In the meantime, Americans are taking matters into their own hands, like in the case of The Non-GMO Project, to eliminate GMOs. This label certifies that a product, even if not organic, is GMO-free:

If you want to know more about this topic, go to www.nongmoproject.com

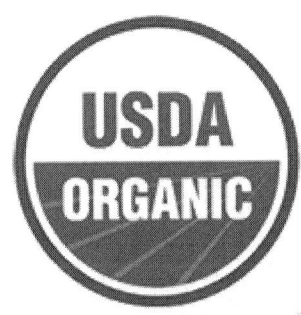

Now let's talk about organic food. The logo above is the only one that certifies organic produce in the US. In order to display this logo, the product has to be verified by a USDA-approved independent agency meeting the following guidelines:

- Abstain from the application of prohibited materials (including synthetic fertilizers, pesticides, and sewage sludge) for three years prior to certification and then continually throughout their organic license.

- Prohibit the use of GMOs and irradiation.

- Employ positive soil building, conservation, manure management, and crop rotation practices.

- Provide outdoor access and pasture for livestock.

- Refrain from antibiotic and hormone use in animals.

- Sustain animals on 100% organic feed.

- Avoid contamination during the processing of organic products.

- Keep records of all operations.

- 95% or more of the ingredients must have been grown or processed without synthetic fertilizers or pesticides and the produce is certified non-GMO.

NOTE: If a label says 'made with organic ingredients', the food must have a minimum of 70% of all its ingredients that meet the above standards.

Here are a few reasons to consider buying certified organic produce:

1. Eating organic helps to reduce the toxins in your body, on the soil, in water and in the air.

2. Organic crops are more nutritious.

Many question the nutritional benefit of organic crops over conventionally grown crops. A recent study[ix] shed new light on the debate, providing evidence that organic foods are richer in nutrients and antioxidants, and lower in heavy metals, especially cadmium and pesticides. Other studies[x] suggest that good soil nutrition increases the production of cancer-fighting compounds called flavonoids, and that conventional farming practices like pesticide and herbicide use disturb their production.

3. Organic produce must be GMO-free.

4. Organic farming is good for the earth, as it preserves our ecosystem.

5. You can't expect to fuel your body and achieve optimal health by eating food laced with toxic chemicals, which your body doesn't recognize.

I know eating 100% organic might not be available where you live or it's not within your budget. This is why I recommend that you either switch to organic or buy verified non-GMO if you consume any of these top GMO foods[xi] and ingredients:

- Soy

- Corn (including high fructose corn syrup, corn oil, corn syrup)

- Sugar beets (most sugar is made from this)

- Canola (as in canola oil)

- Cotton (including cottonseed oil)

- Alfalfa

- Zucchini

- Yellow squash

Papaya

If you want to take it one step further, the Environmental Working Group (EWG), a non-profit that protects human health and the environment, has also created two lists called the Dirty Dozen and the Clean Fifteen to help people who want to reduce their exposure to pesticides when they cannot afford an all-organic diet. You can find the full updated list for 2019 in the next page.

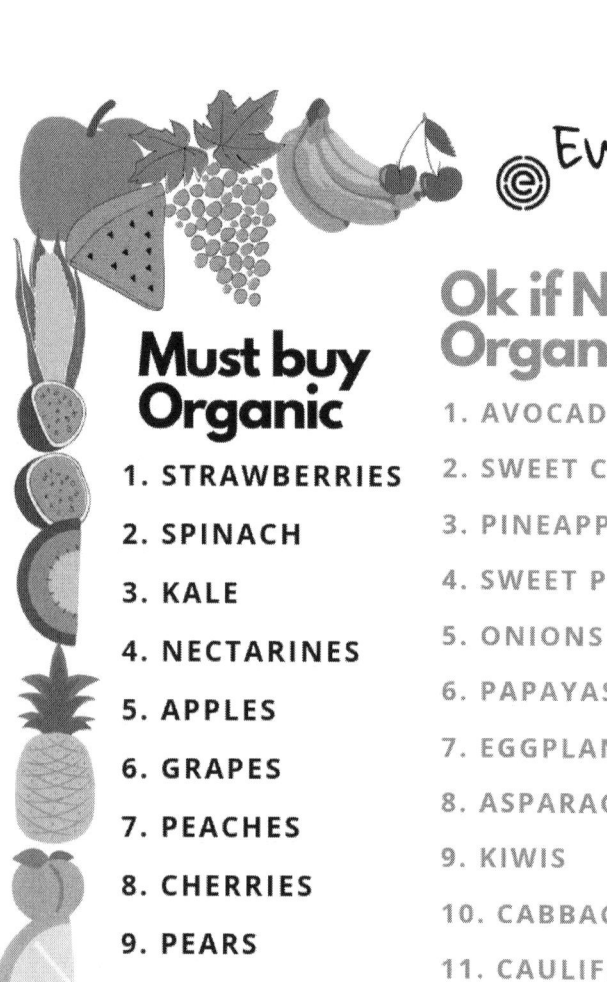

EWG's 2019 List

Must buy Organic

1. STRAWBERRIES
2. SPINACH
3. KALE
4. NECTARINES
5. APPLES
6. GRAPES
7. PEACHES
8. CHERRIES
9. PEARS
10. TOMATOES
11. CELERY
12. POTATOES

Ok if NOT Organic

1. AVOCADOS
2. SWEET CORN
3. PINEAPPLES
4. SWEET PEAS FROZEN
5. ONIONS
6. PAPAYAS
7. EGGPLANTS
8. ASPARAGUS
9. KIWIS
10. CABBAGE
11. CAULIFLOWER
12. CANTALOUPES
13. BROCCOLI
14. MUSHROOMS
15. HONEYDEW MELONS

LEARNING ABOUT LABELS

As our society becomes ever more health-conscious, food manufacturers have wised up and started using misleading words to convince us to buy their products.

Before we get started detoxing our kitchen and pantry, which is going to be your action for this week, let me show you how you have been tricked up to now and why you should ignore any health claims on packaged foods.

THE BIGGEST LABEL SCAMS

Knowing what a food claim truly means is a great way to educate yourself about what you are really eating. When 'organic', 'all natural', 'low fat', 'sugar free', 'zero calorie' and many more have long been a part of popular food vocabulary, it's worth knowing that just because a food is labeled 'natural' doesn't mean it is. That's how these terms often get slapped on food items that may not be healthy at all.

Light: To be considered a 'light' product, the fat content has to be 50% less than the amount found in comparable products. **What's the catch?** There is no regulation to stop manufacturers labeling their product 'light' referring to the flavor, so most of the time, producers still put 'light' on their product although their fat content remains the same.

Multigrain: This sounds very healthy, but basically means that there is more than one type of grain in the product. **What's the catch?** Too bad that most of the time those are processed grains, unless the product is marked as '100% whole grain'.

Whole wheat: Although the idea behind 'whole' can make this label appear healthy, whole wheat means only that they used whole wheat in their ingredients. **What's the catch?** Wheat is known as a trigger for many health issues and I would suggest you eat it cautiously. Look for 'whole grain' instead.

Made with whole grain: Usually, there is very little whole grain in the product. **What's the catch?** Check the ingredients list and look to see if the whole grain is placed in the first three ingredients. If not, then the amount is negligible.

Natural: USDA guidelines state that 'natural' meat and poultry products can only undergo minimal processing and cannot contain artificial colors, flavors, preservatives or other artificial ingredients. **What's the catch?** There are currently no standards for this label for other produce. So a 'natural' cookie simply means that at some point the manufacturer had a natural ingredient to work with.

Organic: If a product has the USDA label that says organic, it is usually a great quality. **What's the catch?** Organic does not equal healthy! When people become more health-conscious, they tend to buy more organic-certified produce. The result is that this label has been slapped onto anything to lead you to think a product is healthy when it is actually not. A brownie, even if labeled 'organic', is still a brownie!

Gluten-free: It simply means that the product doesn't contain wheat, spelt, rye or barley. **What's the catch?** Gluten-free does not equal healthy. Just like the organic label, 'gluten-free' has been abused in order to make you believe certain products are healthier. Many foods that are labeled 'gluten-free' are highly processed and loaded with chemicals, unhealthy fats and sugar. So, for the record, a gluten-free cookie is still a cookie!

No added sugar: Some products are naturally high in sugar and the fact that they don't have added sugar doesn't mean they're healthy. **What's the catch?** Most of the time, unhealthy sugar substitutes may also have been added. Fake sugars create all sorts of issues for your body. (More on sugar in the following week's chapter.)

Sugar-free: These products often contain sugar alcohols, which are lower in calories (roughly 2 calories per gram, compared to 4 per gram for sugar), but compare labels to see if the sugar-free version is any better than the regular version. (Common sugar alcohols are mannitol, xylitol, or sorbitol.)

Lightly sweet or slightly sweetened: Sometimes marketing comes up with their own terms to put on food, which are simply meaningless. These are two examples.

Low–calorie: Low-calorie products have to contain one third fewer calories than the *same* brand's original product. **What's the catch?** A low-calorie version of one brand may contain similar calories as the whole/original product of another brand.

Low-fat: Less than 3g fat per serving. **What's the catch?** Usually serving size is much smaller than you would normally choose. Also, this almost always means that the fat has been reduced at the cost of adding more sugar or chemicals. Be very careful and read the ingredients listed on the back.

Zero trans fat: 'Zero trans fat' actually means less than 0.5 grams of trans fat per serving. So, if a product says zero trans fat on it, it isn't actually at zero. **What's the catch?** Usually the serving sizes are misleadingly small and the product actually contains a lot of trans fat for that portion of food. If the consumer were to have even two servings, then you would get a sizable amount of trans fat by eating it.

Fruit-flavored: Many processed foods have a name that refers to a natural flavor, such as strawberry yogurt. **What's the catch?** There may not be any fruit in the product, only chemicals designed to taste like fruit. Check the label.

Made with real fruit: Products that claim to be made with real fruit may not contain much fruit at all. **What's the catch?** Check the ingredient list and make sure they are not using any 'extract' or 'flavor'. You want to read the fruit name alone without any term attached to it.

Cholesterol-free or low-cholesterol: Cholesterol-free products must contain less than 2 mg per serving while low-cholesterol products can contain 20 mg or less per serving. Foods that say 'reduced' or 'less cholesterol' need to have at least 25% less than comparable products. **What's the catch?** Usually serving size is much smaller than what you would normally buy.

HOW TO OUTSMART LABELS

After you have learned the little scams above, you may agree that reading labels is one tricky business. Have you ever bought a grocery item over another because of the health claims on the label? Well, you may have been conned, but don't worry, you are not alone! In fact, the regulations behind food labeling are complex, and according to a Nielsen survey, nearly 59% of the population has a hard time understanding the true meaning behind them.

Now that you understand the biggest 'tricks' played by manufacturers, it's time to learn a simple process that will help you understand what's really in your food. Become a food detective and investigate what you choose to put into your body. Try these tips when reading labels to sort out the junk from the truly healthy foods:

- **DON'T GET MISLED BY THE CLAIM ON THE FRONT LABEL**

Front labels try to lure you into purchasing products by making health claims. Manufacturers want to make you believe that their product is healthier than other similar options.

- **LOOK AT THE INGREDIENT LIST**

And I don't mean run to the back to read the fat and calories of a product.

Scan the first three ingredients because that is mostly what you're eating. Product ingredients are listed by quantity, from highest amount to lowest amount. The first three listed ingredients are what the producer used most. If you see sugar, oil and some refined grain/flour in the first three ingredients, it's likely that the product is unhealthy. If the ingredients list is longer than two or three lines, or it has more than ten ingredients, you can assume that the product is highly processed. Try to choose items that have whole foods listed as the first three ingredients.

- **WATCH OUT FOR SERVING SIZE**

Manufacturers try to deceive consumers into thinking that their products have fewer calories and less sugar than they really do by displaying nutritional facts for serving size that are often much smaller portions than you would normally eat. Let's take cereals, for example. The nutritional facts often indicated on a label are for a ¾ cup of cereal. Play along with me for a second… Go into the kitchen right now and take out a ¾ cup measuring tool. When do you or your kids ever have that little cereal in your life? If you want to know the real nutritional value of the whole box, you have to multiply the nutritional info given on the back by the 'servings per container' amount on the top right corner.

- **WATCH OUT FOR SUGAR CONTENT!**

Most products contain multiple forms of sugar and sweeteners with different names. There are about 56 names for sugars, as we will see in depth later on, but here are the most common ones you need to watch out for: barley malt, fruit concentrate, beet sugar, brown sugar, buttered syrup, caramel, carob syrup, corn syrup, date sugar, dehydrated cane juice, dextrose, Florida crystals, glucose, golden syrup, high fructose corn syrup, sorbitol, sorghum syrup, sugar, turbinated, xylitol, and anything ending in -ose, which are all sugars.

THE STICKER ON YOUR FOOD

Have you ever wondered about that sticker on your fruits and vegetables? Although they may seem insignificant, those stickers do much more than scanning the price at the checkout stand. In fact, a PLU (price look-up) code can also be a great way to identify if the fruit is GMO, organic or grown conventionally with chemical fertilizers, fungicides, or herbicides.

Here's how:

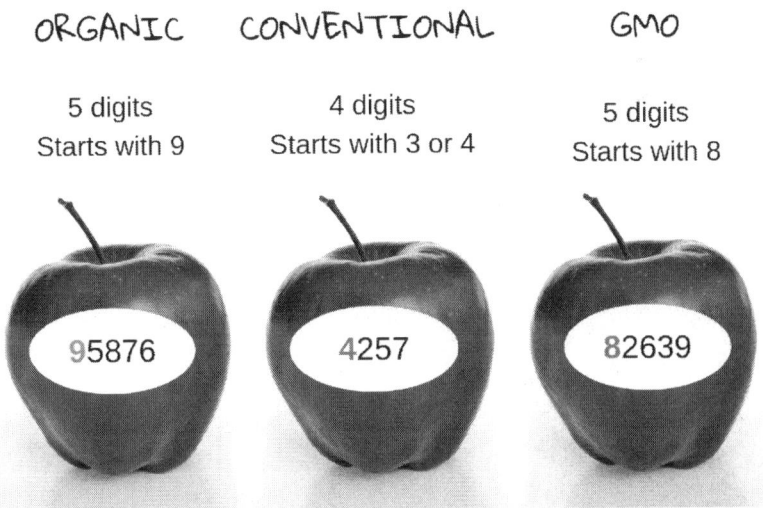

ORGANIC — 5 digits, Starts with 9 — 95876
CONVENTIONAL — 4 digits, Starts with 3 or 4 — 4257
GMO — 5 digits, Starts with 8 — 82639

- **ORGANIC:** *There are five numbers in the code, and the number starts with 9.* As you just learned, organic also means that the product is non-GMO.

- **CONVENTIONAL (grown with the use of pesticides):** *There are only four numbers in the PLU starting with 3 or 4.* The last four letters of the PLU code are simply what kind of vegetable or fruit. An example is that all bananas are labeled with the code of 4257 or 3011.

- **GMO: There are five numbers in the code, and the number starts *with 8.***

Although producers are not obliged to put a PLU sticker on their produce, which gives space for GMO manufacturers to not label theirs, organic and conventional produce are almost always given a code and a label. If not, then keep in mind the most prevalent GMO crops in the US as listed before and make sure to get those organic.

TRY: AVOID HARMFUL CHEMICALS WEEK

In order to detox your life and make space for a new way of living and eating, the first step is to detox your kitchen. This week you'll need to become a food detective, going through all your shelves, drawers and cabinets, and reading all the labels of any packaged food you've relied on up to now.

I know this may sound overwhelming, but avoiding harmful chemicals is a lot easier and more economical than you might think.

I created a cheat sheet on the next page, to help you clear out your fridge and pantry. But let's see how to do it step-by-step.

HARMFUL CHEMICALS

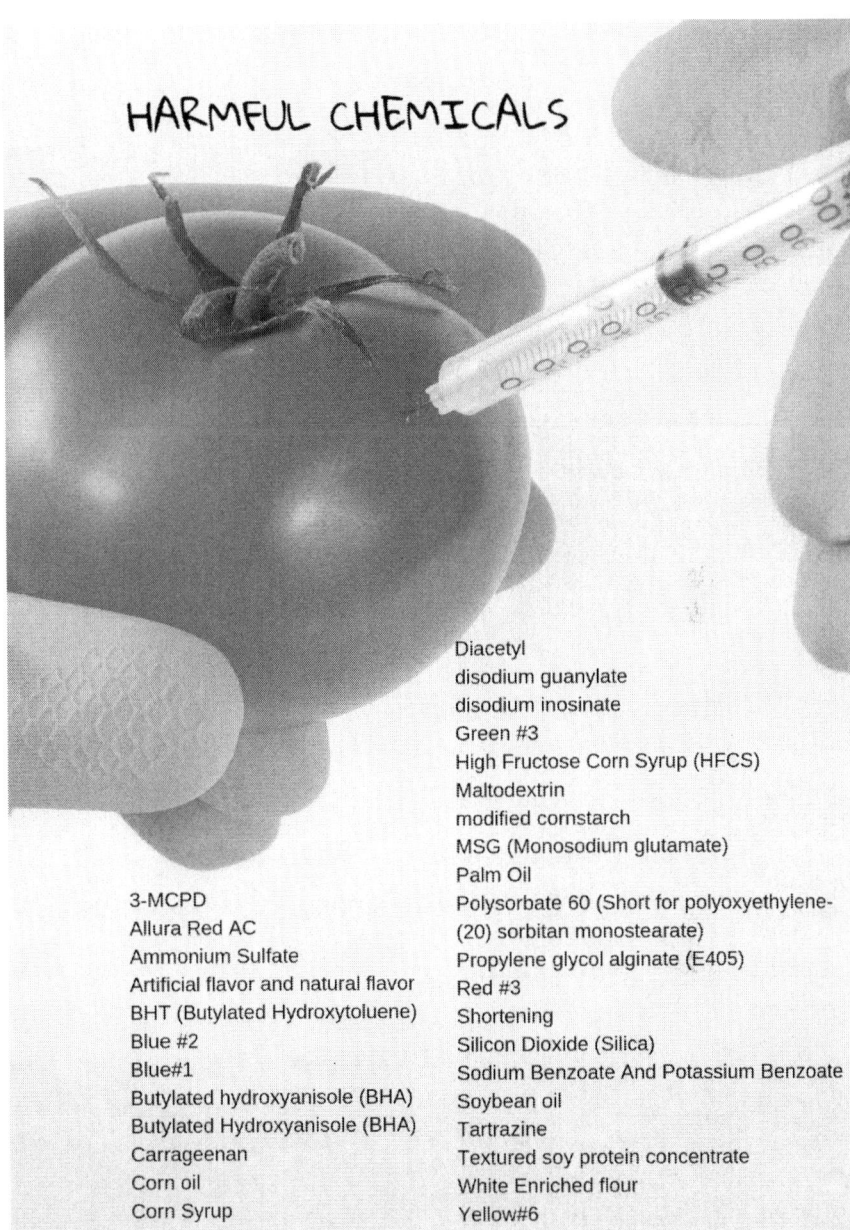

3-MCPD
Allura Red AC
Ammonium Sulfate
Artificial flavor and natural flavor
BHT (Butylated Hydroxytoluene)
Blue #2
Blue#1
Butylated hydroxyanisole (BHA)
Butylated Hydroxyanisole (BHA)
Carrageenan
Corn oil
Corn Syrup

Diacetyl
disodium guanylate
disodium inosinate
Green #3
High Fructose Corn Syrup (HFCS)
Maltodextrin
modified cornstarch
MSG (Monosodium glutamate)
Palm Oil
Polysorbate 60 (Short for polyoxyethylene-
(20) sorbitan monostearate)
Propylene glycol alginate (E405)
Red #3
Shortening
Silicon Dioxide (Silica)
Sodium Benzoate And Potassium Benzoate
Soybean oil
Tartrazine
Textured soy protein concentrate
White Enriched flour
Yellow#6

DETOX YOUR KITCHEN

It's time to put all you have learned into action!

Up to now, your kitchen may have been under the cruel reign of toxins and processed foods, but you can change that right here, right now! A healthy kitchen provides the foundation for a healthy you. If you only fill your kitchen with foods that nourish rather than tempt or harm you, you will automatically make the right choices. By detoxing your kitchen, you will remove all opportunities for sabotaging yourself. If it's not there, you won't eat it. It's that simple. Think about it. If you're craving a cookie, but the only way to eat it is to get in your car and drive a couple of miles, or get out of the house and walk a couple of blocks, it's unlikely you will end up eating a cookie.

So, we're going to start straight away. Time to eliminate all the obstacles to your health and wellness, and transform your kitchen into a place of nourishment and healing! Get excited! Here we go:

Step 1: Set aside three hours to purge the kitchen.

Keep in mind it might take a little longer depending on how much hidden junk and toxins you have in your kitchen. In my experience with my clients, it can take up to three hours to go through everything if you have a big family, but in most cases, you should be done within an hour. A good time-saving trick is to get your family and kids involved. By making a game out of reading the labels and finding the toxic ingredients, you will cut down on the time this process takes and get everyone excited about supporting your journey.

Step 2: Prepare a big garbage bag...

If not two! If you have garbage containers, even better, as the bags may get heavy fast and could break while carrying them out.

Step 3: Read the labels and dump the junk.

I don't believe in dictating to anyone what they should or shouldn't eat. This program was created with the goal of teaching you about food and creating new habits that will help you reach your desired level of health. Ultimately, it's up to you whether or not you remove these foods from your diet, but keep in mind that these foods contain ingredients that impede weight management and may be harmful to your overall health.

Get ready! It's time to go through your fridge, pantry and cabinets, and put what you have learned so far into action. Here comes a list with everything that's gotta go if you want to see real results.

Anything made in a factory that comes in a can, box or package, unless it has only three to five real ingredients: By 'real ingredients', I mean names that a four-year-old could understand, such as 'water' or 'salt'. Sugar should not be one of them. Anything that sounds Latin or you can barely read has to go. Here is a shortlist of common items that you might want to investigate further:

- Crackers
- Canned soups
- Jam
- Cereal
- Rice cakes
- Pre-packaged trail mix
- White pasta
- Tortilla shells
- Wraps
- White bread

- Bagels
- Kraft Dinner
- Pop-Tarts
- Store-bought dressing
- Mayonnaise
- Margarine
- Sauces (barbecue, teriyaki, ketchup)
- Nut butters with added ingredients
- Flavored yogurt
- Processed meats (deli meats, hot dogs, bacon)
- Microwavable dinners
- Fries
- Chicken nuggets
- Processed burgers
- Pizzas
- Pop (diet, iced tea, energy drinks, flavored water)
- Granola bars/protein bars
- All chips (including natural ones)
- Dairy ice cream
- Chocolate (excluding raw cacao bars)
- Candy
- Pre-made muffins
- Donuts

Liquids: These empty calories are often forgotten, but they're the easiest to remove. Switch sugary soft drinks and juices for homemade iced teas and fruit-infused water. Mix up your water with fresh fruits (lemon, lime, and orange slices are my personal favorites) or herbs (such as fresh mint and basil).

Anything that contains hydrogenated oils or refined vegetable oils (corn, peanut, cottonseed and soybean oil): They are most commonly found in fried foods, baked goods, coffee creamers, packaged snacks, margarine, vegetable shortenings, cereal, bread, pasta and sauce mixes, most frozen foods, low-fat ice-creams.

Any food or drink with artificial sweeteners coloring or dyes: The artificial sweeteners are: saccharin, aspartame, acesulfame potassium (Ace-K), sucralose, neotame, dextrose, glucose syrup, crystalline fructose, high fructose corn syrup, fruit juice concentrates, maltodextrin, trehalose, alitame, cyclamates, neohesperidin, thaumatin.

Anything in the fridge that contain any of the above: It's inevitable you will eventually open the fridge looking for something when you are hungry, tired, or stressed, so make sure the choices there are going to help you, not hurt you. Arrange the foods so that the healthiest ones are the most accessible and appealing. Cut up veggies and fruit to keep in little glass containers, stacked for easy access.

Anything in a can that is not labeled 'BPA-free': Many food manufacturers coat the inside of metal cans with a resin made of BPA (bisphenol-A, an endocrine-disrupting chemical), which can leach into foods. Instead, opt for glass jars or frozen foods.

Step 4: Ban plastic and non-stick cookware from the kitchen.

Exposure to certain chemicals found in some plastics (BPA being one) and non-stick cookware (like Teflon and PFOA) have been linked to human health problems including reproductive disorders and cancer. The risk of chemical migration into food increases when plastic or Teflon is damaged or heated. For this reason, I highly recommend you replace the following.

POTS AND PANS: The best pots and pans are stainless steel, cast iron, and ceramic or ceramic-coated. Personally, I use ceramic pots and pans as they are light in weight and naturally non-stick. I understand that replacing cooking pans can be expensive, but it's definitely a good investment for your health. My best suggestion is to shop at HomeGoods and start by replacing one piece at a time. If your current cookware has scratches, especially if made with Teflon, you might want to consider replacing it with something safer ASAP as Teflon or PFCs cause cancer.

KITCHEN UTENSILS: Use silicone, wood, bamboo or stainless-steel, absolutely no plastic, as it leaves chemicals in your food when heated.

BOTTLES: Opt for food-grade stainless steel or glass-lined bottles.

FOOD CONTAINERS: Durable stainless steel and glass are the best containers out there. When using food containers make sure they are BPA-free, lead-free, PVC-free, phthalate-free. And please, don't ever, ever put plastic food containers in the microwave or dishwasher, even if labeled 'microwave safe' or 'dishwasher safe'.

MICROWAVE: I'd like to take a moment to address microwave use, which seriously depletes the nutrients in your food and causes pathological changes in food structure. Once a food's structure is altered, it cannot perform the desired function in your body. Clinical studies show that microwave heating of milk or cooking of vegetables is associated with a decline in hemoglobin levels, which may contribute to anemia, rheumatism, fever, and thyroid deficiency. So please, try to limit the use of your microwave.

Step 5: Organize your kitchen.

Time to take a look around the rest of your kitchen. What would make it easier for you to cook healthy delicious meals and feel good while doing it? The kitchen needs to be your new temple, so how can you honor and improve it? For example, could you:

- Clean out your drawers and cabinets so they are free of clutter?

- Arrange your pots and pans for easier access?

- Make sure you have all the cooking utensils you need? (Make a list of the ones you need to buy.)

- Refresh your supply of spices, condiments, oils, vinegars and sauces so you can cook anything, at any time, without having to run out to the supermarket?

- Find new recipes online or in cookbooks to get the excitement going?

Step 6: Restock your kitchen.

It's grocery time! The part where you get to refill your cabinets and fridge with all the ingredients and foods that will promote your health and wellbeing!

SHOPPING ON A BUDGET

Now that you've cleared out your fridge and cabinets, it's time to restock them with whole, real, fresh foods. I know this topic can be a little bit of a struggle, especially for larger families. Eating well shouldn't and doesn't have to cost an arm and a leg. With the right tips and tricks, you can stick to your budget and even save some cash.

Skip your daily habit

I encourage you to take a detailed look at how much money you spend every week on coffees, sodas, convenience foods and takeouts. Did you know that if you give up that daily latte, you could save almost $1,500 a year? Think what else you could do with that money! By ditching processed foods, you will save money too, especially in the long-term cost of treating diseases that result from eating processed, toxic foods.

Buy in bulk

And create your own portion-controlled packs whenever possible. Seek out local farmers' markets, where you can find fresh produce for less money, or lower-cost stores like Trader Joe's and shopping clubs like Sam's Club or Costco for vegetables, olive oil, fruits, nuts, canned beans and fish.

Skip the pre-prepared, pre-cut foods and DIY

Pre-sliced, pre-cleaned, pre-cut fruits and veggies provide convenience at a higher price. Do it yourself and save some money. Instead of buying mono-serving size packages, buy in bulk and divide it into Ziploc bags yourself.

Buy lesser known brands

Oftentimes, less famous brands (like GreenWise or 365) are better priced than the well-known ones without sacrificing the quality. Check the labels and compare the prices. You may be surprised!

Buy local and in season

While produce is usually available out of season, it's cheaper when it's in season. Take advantage of the savings of seasonal produce by shopping and planning meals with this in mind. For even further savings, go straight to the source and shop at a farmer's market where the produce comes straight from the farmers, eliminating shipping and processing costs. Plus, you'll be supporting local small businesses.

Don't go shopping when hungry

You've heard this one before! It seems like such obvious advice, but a great way to save money at the grocery store is to make sure you don't shop while hungry. If you do, suddenly everything you see becomes something you need or want, and you will probably end up throwing away some, just because you overdo it.

Go prepared

Learn to plan your meals in advance and arm yourself with a list so you'll avoid overspending or buying food that ends up going to waste. Once you get to the store, resist the temptation to buy things not on your list, unless they're items you're substituting that are on sale or cheaper.

Look for sales

Never underestimate the power of sales. You can also shop the sales online. Many grocery stores will post weekly sales and coupons on their website. Foods in the 'bargain bin' so to speak may be close to going bad, so just make sure to adjust your meal plan to eat those items first.

Stick to the outside aisles

Usually, the outside aisles are where you'll find all the fresh produce. By avoiding aisles with frozen meals, chips and chocolate, you will skip the temptation and save some money. You're going to discover there are only a few aisles in the store you actually need to walk down.

By doing this kitchen detox for yourself, you can make your family healthier too. Some members of your tribe may resist at first, but if they shift their eating patterns, even a little, they will feel better.

HEALTHY KITCHEN MUST-HAVES

Now that you've purged unhealthy foods, you'll want to replenish kitchen cabinets and cupboards with fresh, healthy foods. Here is a list of all my kitchen staples and ideas on how to reload your refrigerator and freezer.

Top shelf: Trade out whole milk for milk substitutes like: almond, hemp, cashew and/or coconut milk. Make sure to buy the unsweetened version and watch out for carrageen on the label. Also try replacing the milk you use next time you're baking or cooking.

Refrigerator door: Replace your mayonnaise for vegenaise, the vegan version of mayonnaise. I'm not a vegetarian and I've never been a big fan of fake meats or fake cheeses, but this condiment tastes a hundred times better than mayo, has no additives or preservatives, is lower in saturated fat, and has absolutely no cholesterol. My favorite brand is Follow Your Heart Vegenaise. Also, find a better brand for your ketchup and mustard. I always buy the organic version, Annie's Organic, 365 Organic Ketchup and Trader Joe's Organic are all great options. Chicken broth is another of my favorite condiments; I buy it in resealable cartons and use it to cook rice, mash potatoes or sauté vegetables to enrich the flavor without butter or oil.

Produce bins: Get in the habit of keeping your fridge and freezer stocked with fresh foods. Make sure to fill these bins to the brim with the freshest fruits and vegetables you can find. Here are some ideas for you to try:

- **Non-starchy veggies and salad!** When you can, avoid the most pesticide-contaminated vegetables by consulting the EWG Dirty Dozen list at www.ewg.org to avoid toxins and chemicals.

- **Leafy greens** like spinach, kale, Swiss chard and collards provide an abundance of vitamins, minerals, potassium and calcium. Find a way to incorporate them to your eating habits: add them to smoothies, omelets, soups or healthy flatbreads.

- **Limit fruits** because they increase your insulin levels. Berries are the best fruit out there. Packed with lots of antioxidants, they can be a great for an afternoon snack, a wonderful addition to your smoothie or yogurt, or a healthy dessert. When purchasing fruit, especially if you eat the skin, try always to choose organic to avoid toxins and chemicals. Apples are good options too. In general, Red Delicious and Golden Delicious are your best bargains and they store well in the fridge (for two to four weeks), so don't be afraid to get the bulk bags.

- **Lemons.** Add some lemon to your water, meal or juice to delight your taste buds and help your body detox. This is an absolute must!

- **Avocadoes.** It's one of my favorite staples as it is incredibly versatile. Throw one into a smoothie, spread on toast, smash for guacamole, bake with an egg inside or slice it up in a salad. You can also make a kick-ass chocolate mousse with it in only three minutes. There's a recipe on my website for you to check out.

- **Sweet potatoes.** Make sweet potatoes your new everyday favorite by using them to prepare oven fries, mashed potatoes and stews. Their high fiber content and sweet flavor can also help curb your sweet tooth.

Other Fridge items: Here are some of my other favorite products to always keep in hand:

- **Pre-cut veggies:** Celery, cucumbers, carrots and bell peppers are great for a quick healthy snack. I cut and store them in my fridge so they are that effortless grab-and-go snack.

- **Hummus:** This is the healthiest alternative to processed dips. Make sure to read the ingredient list, because hummus can also often be highly processed. Making your own hummus with fresh chickpeas is always the best option; it only takes a few minutes and is so much tastier than the one you buy at the store.

- **Garlic:** This is a go-to flavor enhancer for just about any dish.

- **Eggs:** A low-cost, high-quality protein source that can help you stay full for longer and reduce your overall food intake. When stored properly in the fridge, raw eggs last about three weeks in the shell. Remember to buy organic, pasture-fed, free-range eggs.

- **Plain/kefir yogurt:** A wholesome, protein and calcium-rich snack, smoothie base or breakfast option. Yogurt can be incredibly healthy, rich in high-quality protein, beneficial probiotics, calcium, B vitamins and even cancer-fighting conjugated linoleic acid (CLA). But be mindful! Most yogurts sold in US grocery stores have a lot of sugar in them, and often hidden. Make sure to read the ingredient list and steer clear of any flavored ones. Instead, make your own variety by adding fresh fruit yourself.

- **Bananas:** Probably one of the best bargains in the fruit department, bananas make a convenient grab-and-go snack, can easily be sliced into cereal or oatmeal, and are great layered on a peanut butter sandwich. They store well in the fridge (one to two weeks). And if they become overripe, peel and toss them in the freezer in a Ziploc for future use in smoothies or baked goods.

- **Fresh proteins (unless vegan):** When selecting beef, meat or poultry, choose grass-fed, hormone-free or organic, whenever possible. If you don't eat them by the second or third day, you can throw them in the freezer for future use.

- **Mushrooms:** Great for detoxifying, as an antioxidant and packed with vitamin D. This simple veggie can help fight cancer, regulate insulin levels and blood pressure, and boost your immunity! Simply sauté with garlic and olive oil for a simple side dish or add them to soups, eggs or burgers.

FREEZER

Frozen vegetables: One of the most valuable items in the grocery store — and just as nutritious frozen as when the veg is fresh.

Frozen spinach: Thaw frozen chopped spinach and eat alone with some olive oil and lemon, or add to anything and everything — from burgers to eggs, tacos to smoothies.

Frozen fruit: If you buy packages of frozen fruit, make sure it has been frozen with no additives. Frozen fruit can be quite pricey so a great alternative to save some money is to buy fresh fruit in bulk during the season and then cut, peel and freeze for the off-season months.

PANTRY

Dry foods: These staple foods usually have a longer shelf life and include raw or lightly roasted nuts and seeds, legumes, quinoa and gluten-free grains.

GRAINS and PASTA

- Oats
- Millet
- Quinoa
- Amaranth

- Brown rice
- Wild Rice
- Quinoa pasta
- Red lentil pasta

NUTS

These are a great snack, easy to carry around and quick addition to any meal!

- Almonds
- Cashews
- Walnuts
- Chestnuts
- Hazelnuts

- Pine nuts
- Pistachios
- Macadamia nuts
- Pecan

SEEDS

Soak some chia overnight to eat as a pudding for breakfast. All of these seeds are a powerhouse of goodness and a nutritious addition to smoothies, salads or soups.

- Chia seeds

- Flax seeds

- Hemp seeds

LEGUMES

Legumes are great unless you are pre-diabetic or diabetic.

- Lentils

- Beans

- Chickpeas

Herbs, spices and seasonings: Herbs and spices are great for adding flavor to your food, reducing your sodium intake and keeping in your store cupboard. They tend to last a long time, so you will get a lot of value out of them. Just read the labels to ensure they don't contain hidden sugar, gluten or other additives. Some of my favorites there are:

- Pink Himalayan salt

- Freshly ground black pepper

- Cumin

- Turmeric

- Curry

- Ground ginger

- Red pepper flakes

- Paprika

- Coconut oil

- Extra virgin olive oil

- Balsamic vinegar
- Bragg's apple cider vinegar

Shelves: When replenishing your pantry and fridge shelves, keep in mind that "out of sight, out of mind" can work against you. If the healthiest foods are hidden in the back of the pantry or refrigerator, you are less likely to eat them. Try to position all the new good stuff where it is always the most easily available.

Miscellaneous for extra detox: Certain foods speed up the process of detoxification and allow more effective and efficient weight loss. The foods that help boost these detox pathways are rich in B vitamins, vitamin A, vitamin C, antioxidants and special detoxifying chemicals called phytonutrients. These are commonly found in:

- Bok choy
- Broccoli
- Brussels sprouts
- Cabbage
- Cauliflower
- Cayenne pepper
- Cilantro
- Collards
- Garlic
- Ginger
- Kale
- Lemon
- Onion
- Parsley
- Rosemary
- Watercress
- Sea vegetables, like wakame, arame, kombu
- Eggs (not a plant food but contain detoxifying nutrients and sulfur)

- Nutritional yeast powder
- Kelp noodles

Superfoods for smoothies: if you want to add extra power to your smoothies have fun with it and experiment with the following:

- Acai berry powder (anti-aging and fat-loss properties)

- Bee pollen (can enhance energy and endurance; great before a workout or when you have low energy)

- Cacao powder

- Chlorella (great detoxifier, boosts immune system, improves focus, improves digestion, increases energy, balances blood sugar and pressure, balances pH, reduces risk of cancer)

- Cinnamon (can be used to help treat muscle spasms, vomiting, diarrhea, infections, the common cold, loss of appetite, and erectile dysfunction (ED); may lower blood sugar in people with Type I or Type II diabetes)

- Maca powder

- Spirulina powder (complete protein source, making it a great addition to anyone's food habits; helps lower inflammation and increase fat-burning during exercise)

- Goji berries (like all berries, high in antioxidants; as research has shown, may offer a huge spectrum of health benefits)

- Unsweetened dry-roasted coconut flakes

Again, you do not need to buy all of these ingredients. These lists are my kitchen staples. I've listed them here to help inspire you with new foods that you may like to add to your selection to kick-start the healthy new you. If you find unfamiliar items among this list, commit to trying one or two each week. You may discover you actually enjoy them!

NOT-SO-HEALTHY FOODS...

I'm not here to tell you that you can't eat these foods, but I'd like to bring some awareness to certain produce that have health disadvantages so that you can make more empowered decisions and help your body achieve optimal health. So, let's look at a few 'healthy foods' you might want to switch for something better next time.

BOXED CEREAL: These are usually full of sugars, toxic ingredients and dyes. Often, they have misleading advertising with very few real health benefits. Stick to oats and chia seeds, and get creative with natural toppings like dried and fresh fruits, nuts and seeds.

PROCESSED MEATS: Any meat that has been modified in order to either improve its taste or extend its shelf life is considered a processed meat. These meats are filled with sodium nitrite (a cancer-causing substance) and other chemicals, flavorings and dyes, which are terrible for your health. No matter what kind of meat you purchase, whether it is shaved or full cut, always try to go to the fresh deli meat counter and skip the pre-packaged versions.

MARGARINE OR FAKE BUTTERS: These products are the unfortunate result of the low-fat diet craze that has seen us ditch healthful fats such as butter for fake varieties. These butter substitutes are highly processed, usually containing trans fats, free radicals, emulsifiers, preservatives, hexane and other solvents. Always stick to real butter!

MICROWAVED POPCORN: Microwave popcorn bags are lined with a compound called PFOA, which when heated, leaches onto the popcorn. The EPA has ruled PFCs as likely carcinogens, and has stated that PFOA "poses developmental and reproductive risks to humans."

ARTIFICIAL SWEETENERS: This topic will be covered in more detail in the next chapter, but for now, just know that studies have found that artificial sweeteners like aspartame can stimulate your appetite, increase carbohydrate cravings, and stimulate fat storage and weight gain.

ANYTHING WITH A HEALTH CLAIM LIKE 'FAT-FREE', 'SUGAR-FREE', 'LOW SUGAR' ON THE LABEL: Usually, these are highly processed or it is unnecessary to follow the advice that the claim aims to promote.

TABLE SALT: Regular table salt and the salt found in processed foods are not the salts that your body needs. They have a large quantity of chemicals added to them and lack the minerals your body actually uses for health. Instead, try Himalayan pink salt or Celtic salt.

PRE-PACKAGED FRUIT OR VEGETABLE JUICES: Usually, these have a high sugar content, and contain added preservatives and chemicals. If you want a juice, make your own.

PRE-MADE SNACKS: 'Lunchables' are just another example of the pre-made snacks to avoid. I know the convenience of opening a snack pack is appealing. Especially ones that say 'only 100 calories' on the label. But when food comes packaged and lasts a long time, it's usually because it is highly processed and includes different chemicals, toxins and unnamed artificial sweeteners. Prepare your own snacks once a week and store them in Ziploc bags or small containers ready to go.

AGAVE: This 'healthy' sweetener is mostly fructose. It is so highly processed and refined that it's better to avoid altogether. Instead, use stevia, raw unfiltered honey or raw sugar, but absolutely not the white kind, which is bleached.

ENHANCED WATER: Flavored water, 'zero calorie' water, 'vitamin' water and so-called 'enhanced' or 'functional' water products all sound like nothing more than flavored water with added vitamins or minerals. Beware! When you start investigating the lists of ingredients, you'll realize you're doing your body more harm than good by falling for this healthy illusion. We will see this in more detail in the next chapter.

SPORT DRINKS: Sports drinks are no different than enhanced water. Most sports drinks are in fact loaded with high fructose corn syrup, sodium, artificial colors and flavors. A far better alternative is coconut water, which has a long list of beneficial nutritional compounds including natural electrolytes, enzymes, trace elements, amino acids, and antioxidants. Coconut water also has anti-inflammatory and blood-pressure-lowering properties, making it the perfect 'sports drink'. **BE AWARE:** Even coconut water contains a lot of sugar and should be limited to when you need to replace minerals and fluid, like after a sauna or long duration cardio, not as a regular water substitute.

ENERGY BARS: Snack bars, health bars, nutrition bars, protein bars, energy bars or meal replacement bars — no matter what you call them, most of them are less healthy than a candy bar and oftentimes more expensive. The majority of commercial energy bars are made with cheap soy protein, high fructose corn syrup, synthetic vitamins and sugars, and waste products from industrial food production.

GLUTEN-FREE SNACK FOODS: Companies are taking advantage of the prevalence of 'gluten-free' talk these days, banking on consumers equating gluten-free with 'healthy'. At the end of the day, gluten-free cookies and crackers are still processed. If you can't do gluten, try making your own snacks so you can omit unwanted additives.

BOTTOM LINE: I'm not here to crucify all processed food. In some cases, some food processing is beneficial to help neutralize the natural toxins in food before it is consumed. And why not? Here and there, it can be a convenient solution when you are in a rush. However, if you consume highly processed foods on a daily basis, your overall health and wellbeing are at risk, and you are more prone to develop diseases. If you can make 90% of your food whole, natural and fresh and just 10% of your meals processed and convenience, it will go a long way toward avoiding all the health issues we have seen. And if once in a blue moon you crave a specific candy bar or something you now know is highly processed, use it as a reward or treat and make it worth your while.

CHECK-IN QUESTIONS

How were your energy levels on a scale of 1 to 10?

Did you feel fatigued or sluggish?

Can you think clearly?

Did you feel tired?

Did you feel bloated?

Did you have headaches? (If yes, how many?)

Did you go to the bathroom regularly?

Is your skin clear?

Did you have cravings?

Did you binge?

Did you eat or snack compulsively or mindlessly?

Is your sleep regular?

Did you have trouble concentrating or brain fog?

Did you suffer with mood swings?

Did you ever feel anxious, fearful, or nervous?

Did you feel physically weak?

Did you get sick?

Did you have bad breath?

Did you have heartburn?

Did you have stomach or intestinal pain?

Did you experience ringing in your ears?

Did you feel the need to urinate urgently or frequently?

Did you have pain or aches in your muscles and joints?

Did you feel stiff or limited in your movements?

"My protein shake brings all the boys to the yard, and they're like: 'damn your muscle are hard.' Damn right! My muscle are hard. I can teach ya, but I'd have to charge."

WEEK 4

ARE PROTEINS THE SECRET TO HEALTHY WEIGHT LOSS?

Welcome to week four, where we'll be turning our attention to protein. Remember to check in with yourself on how you're feeling so far with the changes you've already made. Before reading this section, let me be clear that my views here are not related to the moral ethics of a vegan diet. Instead, the information on the following pages is disclosed on a nutritional, human health basis.

WHY ARE PROTEINS IMPORTANT?

Without protein, life as we know it would not be possible. Our bodies are physically made out of the amino acids from proteins, some of which we can only get from our food, which is why they are called essential amino acids.

Proteins are the main building blocks of the body; they compose muscles, tendons, organs, and skin, and we require them to continuously renew and replenish our cells, stabilize our blood sugar, and be energized.

As such, you can understand how important they are as a part of your health journey. Many foods contain protein, but the richest sources include animal products like meat, dairy, eggs, and fish, as well as some plant sources like beans, nuts, and seeds.

Learning how much protein you need is the next step toward helping your body detoxify and remain healthy and strong. Luckily, your body gives off clear signs when you are consuming too much or too little protein. If you are not getting enough protein, you could experience:

- Strong sugar and sweet cravings

- Inability to concentrate

- Fatigue or 'spacey' feelings

- Anemia

- Hair loss

- Unhealthy facial coloring

On the other hand, if you are consuming too much protein, you could experience symptoms like:

- Low energy

- Constipation

- Tight or stiff joints

- Kidney disease

- Stress

- Bad body odor and bad breath

- Dehydration

- Weight gain

It has been estimated that the right amount of protein for a semi-sedentary person should be between **0.36 to 0.6 grams per pound**[xii]. This amounts to:

- 56-91 grams per day for the average male

- 46-75 grams per day for the average female

To make it simple, with every meal, males should eat a portion of protein the size of two palms of their hands and as thick, while females only one palm size and as thick. That said, just like with fats, eating protein is not just about quantity, but quality as well.

BEST SOURCES OF PROTEIN

Animal protein sources are considered the best sources of essential amino acids, although it is possible to combine plant-based foods.

VEGAN or VEGETARIAN: Most people believe that protein only comes from meat and dairy sources and so they overindulge in these two food groups. Fortunately, meat and dairy are not the only options.

Here are some of my favorite vegan protein sources:

- Quinoa
- Barley

- Black beans
- Brown rice
- Bulgur
- Buckwheat
- Chickpeas
- Peas
- Potatoes
- Lentils

- Kale
- Cauliflower
- Collard greens
- Green beans
- Broccoli
- Brussels sprouts
- Spinach

Additionally, you can also try to get protein from nuts and seeds like:

- Almonds, cashews, and pistachios
- Chia seeds
- Flax seeds

- Hemp hearts / seeds
- Chlorella
- Spirulina
- Sunflower seeds

This list gives only a fraction of your options. Please keep in mind that if you are following an all-vegan or all-vegetarian diet, in order to meet the minimum requirements of proteins, you have to consume a larger and more varied mix of the sources listed here. Hemp is the most complete form of protein for people following a vegan diet. This said, if you follow these types of diets, I highly recommend integrating a vegan protein supplement to make sure you reach your recommended daily dose.

CHICKEN and TURKEY: When it comes to eating meat, white meat is by far your best option, especially if you are trying to detox. I recommend *only organic pasture-raised chickens*, since non-medical use of antibiotics is not permitted in organic farming. Not only are these products safer, but they have a superior nutritional profile as well. Look for the **USDA Organic seal.** Another alternative is to buy chicken directly from your *local farmer or farmers' market*. Just make sure they've been pasture-raised according to organic principles, even if the farmer is not organic certified.

FISH: Fish is one of the greatest sources of protein and healthy fats in the animal world, but as the levels of pollution in our waters have increased, you have to be very picky about which types of seafood you decide to eat. If you're not careful, the toxic effects from the pollutants in the fish, like mercury, arsenic, and PCBs, will outweigh the benefits. A general rule is that the bigger the fish, the higher the chance of contamination. When purchasing fish, just like with everything else, it's always best to buy the highest quality possible, and always favor wild-caught over the farm-raised kind. About half of the world's seafood comes from fish farms, including in the US. Farm-raised fish are generally treated with antibiotics to fend off the germs caused by fish waste and uneaten feed that litter the sea floor beneath these farms. They're also given hormones to make them grow bigger faster. Here are some labels that can help you make your selection:

- **Whole Foods Market Responsibly Farmed:** Third party certification.

- **FishWise:** This label identifies how the fish was caught, where it came from, and whether the fish is sustainable (or environmentally threatened).

- **Seafood Safe:** The Seafood Safe label involves independent testing of fish for contaminants, including mercury and PCBs, and recommendations for consumption based upon the findings.

Wild-caught Alaskan and sockeye salmon are always a great pick but keep yourself informed with the latest news on seafood. There are shopping guides available from the Environmental Defense Fund (edf.org) and Monterey Bay Aquarium (montereybayaquarium.org) that are worth checking to keep you and your family safe and healthy.

MEAT: You may want to consider limiting the amount of red meat you consume to a maximum of four times per month. You may already be aware of the health risk related to beef, but let me remind you why you might want to reconsider your red meat consumption:

- Beef, lamb, and veal are the most contaminated types of meat out there.

- Red meat contains carnitine, which can contribute to heart disease.

- Bacon, hot dogs, and deli meats are sprayed with ammonia, which you ingest.

- Conventionally raised farm animals are pumped full of antibiotics and hormones, which will weaken your immune system.

- Red meat causes inflammation in your body.

If you don't want to eliminate it completely from your diet (I personally still eat red meat every now and then), there are a few actions you need to take to help mitigate the negative health consequences:

1. Purchase organic, grass-fed meat.

2. Consume a highly alkalizing diet to help counter the acidic effects of meat.

3. Use proper serving sizes. The recommended serving size of red meat is the size of a deck of cards. Try your best to only eat this amount.

4. Take a digestive enzyme with HCl before your meal.

Only 30% of the population can excel on a purely plant-based eating regimen. The majority of individuals thrive on a diet that contains a low quantity of red and white meat. To figure out what's best for you, I encourage you to eliminate meat for three weeks and see how you feel. If you feel less energized and 'not yourself', you may need meat in order to thrive, so reintroduce it to your diet, following the tips above.

SOY

Contrary to popular belief, soy is not necessarily a healthful food. Although fermented soy has many beneficial properties, **unfermented soy can get you in trouble**. Unfortunately, most of us eat the type of soy that is not fermented. Rather, we consume unfermented soy in the form of tofu, soy protein isolates (in bars and shake powders), soymilk, fresh, raw, or cooked soybeans, soy chips, soy flour, and countless processed foods that contain soy derivatives or soybean oil. I recommend avoiding all soy products unless they're fermented or sprouted.

But what's so bad about unfermented soy?

- Soy contains high levels of toxins or anti-nutrients that can cause gastric distress.

- Soy contains hemagglutinin that promotes unwanted blood-clotting.

- Soy contains phytates that lead to a mineral deficiency, especially if you are a vegetarian.

- Soy contains goitrogens that can impact your thyroid function.

- Soy contains phytoestrogens that can mimic and even block estrogen.

- Soy is largely genetically engineered. A full 91% of the soy planted in the US is genetically bioengineered to survive heavy application of Monsanto's toxic herbicide.

So, if you can, avoid tofu, soy protein products, and soymilk. Fermented soy (tempeh, natto, soy sauce, miso, and soybean sprouts) are safe to consume as they don't have the above issues. Just make sure they're not pasteurized and that your protein shakes do not contain any unfermented soy. Visit www.mercola.com to learn more about the studies conducted on this topic and the results.

TRY: ADD PROTEINS WEEK

Now that you have a clearer idea on what proteins do, why they are important, and how to source the best ones, it's time to put into action what you have learned. From this point forward, I invite you to add proteins to every meal or snack you have during the day. By doing so, you will help your body sustain energy during the day, curb your cravings, stabilize blood sugar, and allow your body to reach its regular body weight faster.

BOTTOM LINE: Protein is an essential macronutrient that serves many functions in the body. Research shows that high-protein diets also help with weight loss. That said, not all high-protein foods are equal and sourcing protein correctly will ensure you get the benefit rather than increasing toxicity in the body. The simplest way to increase your protein intake is to eat high-protein foods

CHECK-IN QUESTIONS

How were your energy levels on a scale of 1 to 10?

Did you feel fatigued or sluggish?

Can you think clearly?

Did you feel tired?

Did you feel bloated?

Did you have headaches? (If yes, how many?)

Did you go to the bathroom regularly?

Is your skin clear?

Did you have cravings?

Did you binge?

Did you eat or snack compulsively or mindlessly?

Is your sleep regular?

Did you have trouble concentrating or brain fog?

Did you suffer with mood swings?

Did you ever feel anxious, fearful, or nervous?

Did you feel physically weak?

Did you get sick?

Did you have bad breath?

Did you have heartburn?

Did you have stomach or intestinal pain?

Did you experience ringing in your ears?

Did you feel the need to urinate urgently or frequently?

Did you have pain or aches in your muscles and joints?

Did you feel stiff or limited in your movements?

"No need to sugar coat it, you are not Willy Wonka."

WEEK 5

SUGAR:

THE UNSWEETENED TRUTH

There's no getting around it, our generation has a sweet tooth. But did you know that most people eat the equivalent of 30 teaspoons of sugar a day?! Reducing your sugar and sweetener intake will be a huge step towards reaching your body's ideal shape, easing the stress on your liver, and detoxing your body.

We tend to think that sugar is mainly found in sweet foods and desserts like cookies and cakes. Unfortunately, it is commonly also added to many savory foods, most of which you would never imagine contain sugar, such as bread, milk, burgers, and pasta sauce.

This week, we will learn all there is to know about sugar, how it impacts your health, and how reading the labels of what you eat will make you a sugar detective who's ready for anything. Let's get started!

We all know sugar is bad for you, but let's take a moment to understand why, and especially the reasons for eliminating it from your food habits.

Excessive sugar intake can lead to Type II diabetes, contribute to metabolic syndrome, and lead to excessive weight gain. More dangers of consuming sugar include:

- Feeding candida
- Promoting wrinkles and aging skin
- Making your blood acidic
- Potentially leading to osteoporosis
- Rotting your teeth
- Raising your blood-sugar level
- Contributing to obesity
- Addiction (almost as much as drugs)
- Creating the urge to binge
- Providing 'empty calories' with no nutritional value
- Contributing to diabetes
- Robbing your body of minerals
- Robbing you of energy
- Contributing to heart problems
- Potentially causing cancer
- Contributing to ulcers
- Potentially causing gallstones
- Contributing to adrenal fatigue
- Potentially suppressing your immune system
- Raising the level of neurotransmitters called serotonin
- Weakening eyesight

- Potentially causing hypoglycemia (low blood-sugar levels)
- Potentially causing aging
- Potentially contributing to eczema

- Potentially causing arthritis

And not only these but…

TOO MUCH SUGAR WILL MAKE YOU STUPID

As if all this was not enough, recent studies show that too much sugar will affect your brain. A UCLA study[xiii] shows how a steady diet that is high in fructose can damage your memory and learning. To learn more about this research, search for: 'too much sugar will make you stupid'.

Saying this isn't meant to scare you, though. Ironically, your body cannot function properly without sugar, so first, understand that not all sugar is created equal.

As I've said before, you can think of sugar like gas for your car. As there are different kinds of gas, there are also different types of sugars. Each one gets treated by and behaves differently within your body. The major difference is between natural sugars and processed sugars.

Natural sugars are sugars found in nature. These include the naturally occurring sugars found in fruits, veggies, and honey. Foods with natural sugar have an important role in our diet, as they provide essential nutrients that keep the body healthy and help prevent disease.

Processed or artificial sugars are natural sugars that are modified, combined and processed by us humans to create something that tastes sweet but maintains the same texture and consistency. Artificial sweeteners are added to about 6,000 different beverages, snacks, and food products, making label-reading an ever-pressing necessity. Today, all products that claim to have less or no sugar are usually sweetened with artificial sweeteners.

As we've seen, how the body metabolizes something found in nature (such as natural sugars) differs from how it metabolizes something chemically produced (such as refined sugars added to processed foods). The body breaks down processed sugars rapidly, causing insulin and blood-sugar levels to skyrocket, and that's what gets us in trouble. Because refined sugar digests quickly, you also don't feel full after you've eaten, which leads to an overconsumption of food.

There is one last problem that sugar causes in the body. Once sugar passes through the stomach and reaches the small intestine, it doesn't matter if it came from an apple or a soft drink. How much sugar is already in your blood will determine how the body will use it! If you already have a lot of sugar in your system, what you just digested will be stored as fat rather than being used for quick energy and it won't matter whether the sugar comes from junk food or fruit.

THE 61 NAMES OF SUGAR

Disturbingly, food industry manufacturers are trying to hide the presence of sugars and artificial sweeteners in our food, so you may not be aware of the amount of sugar you are actually consuming daily. In fact, added sugar comes in many forms, which is why it's so hard to find on ingredients labels. There are at least 61 different types of sugar used to sweeten our food. Pretty crazy, right?

You can find the full list at the end of this chapter.

It has been estimated that 74% of packaged savory foods sold in supermarkets have added sugars. So, even if you skip dessert, you may still be consuming more sugar than is recommended. In fact, studies show that the average American consumes 22 teaspoons of sugar a day (32 for teenagers), twice the highest amount recommended by the FDA, which urges us to take in no more than 10 teaspoons (6 for women).

What's even scarier is that food manufacturers are not required to notify you if a product contains added sugars, so you need to check the ingredient list carefully. And, as usual, there are schemes played on you here too. For a start, if manufacturers want to sweeten up a certain product, instead of using 15g of sugar (and having to list '15 grams of sugar' on the nutritional label), they will use artificial sugars, so they do not have to. Additionally, manufacturers will trick you by using different types of added sugars so that the amount of each one they use is smaller. For example, they are allowed to say 5g 'malt syrup', 5g 'invert sugar' and 5g 'maltose'. This way, by dividing the total amount of added sugars into three or four different sugar derivates, the names of all the added sugars appear further down the list of ingredients (because the product ingredients are listed in order of weight; the lower the ingredient weight in a product, the lower the rank on the ingredient list). See the catch?

Now that you understand this, you will be surprised to discover that most foods promoted as 'natural' or 'healthy' are actually laden with added sugars. Snack bars or protein bars are a great example of this. When reading the nutritional facts label, they might have a low to 0g of sugars per serving, but when reading the ingredients list you might find out that there are many different added sugars.

WHY ARE WE ADDICTED?

Junk food and sugar flood the reward system with dopamine, particularly in the brain area that is strongly implicated in *addiction*. Sugar also affects opioid pathways within the brain, the same system manipulated by drugs like heroin and morphine. Sugar has a drug-like effect on us, because it releases the neurotransmitter serotonin, giving us a happy, content feeling. Ultimately, the less refined sugar you consume, the less stress your body has to deal with, and the less likely you'll be to ever develop serious diseases like Type II diabetes. The more sugar you eat, especially if you are overweight, the more resistant you become to its impact and the more sugar it takes to set off the reward bells in your brain. This is quite literally the insulin resistance that underpins diabetes. And it can get worse...

WHAT THE HECK IS CANDIDA?

If you consume too much sugar or refined carbs (bread, pasta, and so on) over an extended period of time, you may cause candida to overgrow in your gut. Candida is a fungus (form of yeast) that everyone has in their mouths and intestines. Its main job is to help out with digestion and nutrient absorption, but when overproduced, it can break down the wall of the intestine and penetrate the bloodstream, releasing toxic by-products into your body and causing the infamous 'leaky gut'.

The healthy bacteria in your gut typically keep your candida levels in check. However, a few factors can cause the candida population to grow out of control like:

- Eating a diet high in refined carbohydrates and sugar

- Consuming a lot of alcohol

- Taking oral contraceptives

- Eating a diet high in fermented foods (like kombucha, sauerkraut, and pickles)

- Living a high-stress lifestyle

- Taking a round of antibiotics that killed too many of those friendly bacteria

When the friendly bacteria in your intestines are weakened or damaged, they can't metabolize sugar properly, which cause the 'bad' bacteria (candida) to overgrow. Rice University researchers estimate that 70% of Americans have this systemic fungal infection. That includes men, who also suffer from this condition (AKA candidiasis). It can spread throughout the body and affect the organs as it travels through the bloodstream.

WHY FERMENTED FOODS DO MORE HARM THAN GOOD

While it's true that fermented foods can have health benefits, if you suffer with candida, they may actually cause more harm than good. The fermentation process makes these foods high in yeast and bad bacteria. Not only that, but all of the prebiotics produced during the fermentation process *feed* not only the 'good' bacteria, but the yeast and bad bacteria too.

If you are dealing with candida overgrowth, and already have an overpopulation of yeast or bad bacteria, eating fermented foods is the equivalent of adding fuel to the fire. For this reason, if you think you have candida overgrowth, I recommend avoiding these foods, until your candida is back in check:

- Beer
- Champagne
- Kefir
- Kimchi
- Kombucha

- Sauerkraut
- Vinegar
- Wine
- Yogurt

DO YOU HAVE IT?

To find out if you have candida, there are a couple of ways you can go about it. You can speak to your health practitioner and ask to have a blood test done. There are three antibodies that should be tested to measure your immune system's response to candida – IgG, IgA, and IgM. High levels of these antibodies indicate that an overgrowth of candida is present.

Another way is by a urine tartaric acid test, which detects the waste product of candida yeast overgrowth. An elevated tartaric level means an overgrowth of candida.

Lastly, you can self-test. There are a couple of at home-test kits, and after some research Candidasure seems to be the most accurate.

The most common symptoms of candida are:

- Abdominal pain
- Headaches
- Bad breath
- Rectal itching
- Mood swings
- Memory loss
- Depression
- Acne
- Sinus problems
- PMS
- Vaginitis
- Irritable bowel syndrome (IBS)
- Bladder infections
- Thrush

More symptoms are:

- Skin and nail fungal infections, such as athlete's foot or toenail fungus

- Feeling tired and worn down

- Suffering from chronic fatigue or fibromyalgia

- Digestive issues such as bloating, constipation, or diarrhea

- Autoimmune diseases such as Hashimoto's thyroiditis, rheumatoid arthritis, ulcerative colitis, lupus, psoriasis, scleroderma, or multiple sclerosis

- Difficulty concentrating, poor memory, lack of focus, ADD, ADHD, and brain fog

- Skin issues like eczema, psoriasis, hives, and rashes

- Irritability, mood swings, anxiety, or depression

- Vaginal infections, urinary tract infections, rectal itching, or vaginal itching

- Severe seasonal allergies or itchy ears

- Strong sugar and refined carb (bread, pasta, etc.) cravings

If you suffer with any of the above, I highly recommend you investigate further and get tested for candida. If not healed in time, this little fungus releases toxins that can further weaken your immune system, leading to more serious health problems.

HOW DO YOU GET RID OF IT?

If you tested positive to candida, it's time to take action! As said before, candida is a naturally occurring bacterium in the gut and mouth, so you will never be able to eliminate it completely. You can, however, get it back in check. To do so, you need to do three things:

1. Stop the yeast overgrowth

2. Build up the friendly bacteria

3. Repair your gut so that candida can no longer enter your bloodstream

1. Stop the candida overgrowth.

This mainly requires switching to a low-carb diet. Sugar is what feeds yeast, so step one is to eliminate sugar in all of its simple forms such as candy, desserts, alcohol, and flours. And limit complex carbohydrates, like grains, beans, fruit, bread, pasta, or potatoes, to just one cup a day. This will help prevent the candida from growing further. Also try to eliminate all fermented foods. While it's common knowledge that fermented foods help to feed the good bacteria, most people don't realize that bad bacteria feed off of these foods as well.

Using diet alone could take three to six months before the candida is back under control. To keep this nasty critter from getting out of hand, consider going to see a homeopath to help speed up the process with natural remedies. Meanwhile, also try to avoid the following:

- All dietary sugar (including honey, maple syrup, and refined sugar)

- Alcohol

- Cheese

- Dried fruits (which have a high sugar content)

- Peanuts

- Baked goods

- Raw mushrooms

- Sprouts

- Vinegar

- Gluten-containing grains (wheat, oats, spelt, rye, and barley)

You can also take a supplement of caprylic acid. Caprylic acid comes from coconut oil and basically 'pokes holes' in the yeast cell wall, causing it to die. For a more invasive but quick result, you can also ask your health practitioner about using an anti-fungal medication, such as Diflucan or Nystatin.

2. Rebuild the good bacteria in your gut.

Typically, this is what keeps your candida population under control. Taking anywhere from 50 to 100 billion units of probiotics on a regular basis should help to reduce the candida levels and restore your levels of good bacteria. Also, foods that help heal your gut including garlic, coconut oil, apple cider vinegar (the only vinegar allowed), ginger, cruciferous vegetables, olive oil, cloves, cinnamon, salmon, lemon. Try to avoid conventionally produced animal products such as meats, chicken, and dairy as they may contain antibiotics. Choose organically raised and produced animal products only, which are not given antibiotics.

3. Repair.

Providing the nutrients necessary to help the gut repair itself is essential. L-glutamine, an amino acid that helps to rejuvenate the gut wall lining, is one of my favorite supplements. Other key nutrients include zinc, omega-3 fish oils, vitamins A, C, and E, as well as herbs such as slippery elm and aloe vera.

WHAT'S THE DEAL WITH FRUIT?

There's no doubt that eating fruit is important for our overall health and wellbeing. Mother Nature clearly intended us to eat fruit, but like everything else, too much of a good thing can be bad. And fruit is just another example of this.

Fruit is often praised for its health benefits as it provides us with vitamins, minerals, fiber, antioxidants, and other phytonutrients that are great for our health and help us reduce the risk of disease. But if you are trying to detox or lose weight, too much fruit could sabotage your efforts because fructose turns on your 'fat switch', so to speak.

The key is to understand how glucose and fructose, the two sugars found in fruit, get metabolized by the body. While every cell in the body can use glucose as a form of energy, fructose is metabolized in the liver as opposed to the bloodstream. So, if you eat a lot of fruit and your liver does not need the energy that comes with consuming fructose, it will save the excess for a later time, storing it as fat and sending it to our fat cells. On top of that, researchers believe that 35% of people cannot digest and absorb large amounts of fructose[xiv].

FIVE SIGNS YOU MIGHT BE EATING TOO MUCH FRUIT

If you are experiencing any of these signs, you might want to rethink your sugar consumption:

- **You can't lose weight:** If you have been on a whole food diet for a while, you've cut out soda, candy, and processed foods, but are still not losing weight, you might want to consider looking at your fruit intake. In a recent book called *The Fat Switch*, Dr. Richard Johnson explains how fructose turns your body into a fat-storage machine by turning on your 'fat switch'. His research showed that fructose activates a key enzyme, fructokinase, which activates another enzyme that causes cells to accumulate fat. Interestingly, this is the exact same 'switch' animals use to fatten up in the fall and burn fat during the winter. I know it's unfair to single out fruit, but if you've already overhauled your diet, this could be the missing piece of the puzzle.
- **You're frequently bloated or have diarrhea** Fruit is a

classic trigger for bloating because it is rich in fructose. Unfortunately, this can commonly lead to diarrhea.

- **You suffer with IBS** Many fruits (like apples) are also rich in pectin, a type of fiber that people with IBS may have trouble fully breaking down.
- **You always crave sugar** Not only does eating fruit spike your blood sugar, but it also doesn't sustain it for very long. So, if you have fruit by itself as a snack, you might notice that you're satisfied for 30 minutes or so, but soon after, your tummy starts growling. That's because fruit doesn't have much protein or fat to keep us satisfied for long. The amount of fiber in fruit is not enough to prevent a crash in blood sugar after eating fruit. *What happens then?* We get hungry and we get cravings for foods that will quickly raise the blood sugar — anything sweet or starchy.
- **You are addicted to smoothies and juices** Veggie juice is fine, but juicing fruit strips most of its fiber, creating a huge sugar surge. When the fiber breaks down, the remaining sugar is absorbed rapidly into your bloodstream leading to no weight loss and sugar cravings, as described above. Likewise, when your Vitamix gets to work and mechanically breaks up the cellular structure of the fiber, your body has more immediate access to the sugars contained in the smoothie.

NO, YOU DON'T HAVE TO GIVE UP FRUIT FOREVER

Don't panic! I'm not saying that you should *completely* eliminate fruit from your diet. All I am suggesting is that the idea of eating an unlimited amount of fruit "because it's healthy" should be eliminated, especially if you identify with any of the five signs described above.

Learning how to incorporate fruit properly into your eating regimen will lessen digestive problems, give you tons more energy, and allow you to enjoy all the powerful benefits that come with it. Here is how:

- **The best time to eat fruit is either first thing in the morning on an empty stomach or as a mid-morning snack.**

- **Protein and healthy fat can help buffer fruits' sugar impact.** If you have apple slices, smear a tablespoon of almond butter onto them, or eat those berries with some Greek yogurt. **BE AWARE:** Pre-packed yogurt at the grocery store has very little fruit in it, but tons of sugar, so please buy real fruit and add it to your yogurt!

- **Leave a gap of at least 30 minutes between a meal and a fruit snack.**

Some of my favorite fruits that you could consider keeping around are:

- **Berries:** Make sure to buy wild or organic, as commercially grown berries are bad news. Berries put less stress on your blood-sugar-regulating mechanisms, and provide loads of fiber, vitamins, minerals, and phytochemicals that protect you against disease.

- **Avocados:** These are an excellent source of good fat, fiber, vitamins, and minerals. The fatty acids found in avocados provide excellent fuel for energy.

- **Figs:** These are the most mineral-dense fruit out there, particularly high in potassium, calcium, and iron. Fresh figs are superior to dried figs, so if you are going to eat dried figs, strive to eat only a few.

- **Pomegranates:** A great choice to provide your body with super protection against free radical damage and chronic disease, pomegranates have one of the highest concentrations of antioxidants among all fruits.

- **Apples:** From a practical viewpoint, apples are one of the most affordable healthy fruits to eat on a regular basis. Like all of the fruits listed above, they are high in fiber, vitamins, minerals, and antioxidants.

Again, remember balance is key and everyone is different. If you know you cannot tolerate fruit, or don't normally consume it, don't eat it! Trust your body.

ARTIFICIAL SWEETENERS

Since it's becoming common knowledge that eating sugar-sweetened foods and beverages will cause a number of negative potential health effects, including weight gain or even obesity, Type II diabetes, and metabolic syndrome, many people have switched to non-caloric sweeteners (such as saccharin, aspartame, and sucralose) as less damaging alternatives to sugar. Let's dive into the topic of artificial sweeteners to see what's what.

In the last several years, many people have switched from regular to 'diet' versions of the same product, started checking the labels on other foods and beverages to make sure they are made with sugar substitutes. But are sweeteners healthier or safe?

The answer is no.

There are five dangerous sugar substitutes that are approved for consumer use: saccharin, neotame, acesulfame potassium, aspartame, and sucralose. Of the five main artificial sweeteners, sucralose (Splenda) and aspartame (NutraSweet and Equal) are the most pervasive and dangerous substitutes found in products on store shelves today.

Many studies in the past couple of years have shown how artificial sweeteners may play a role in making worse the very conditions that they are meant to address[xv].

In animals[xvi], artificial sweeteners like sucralose, saccharin, and aspartame have been associated with an increased risk of cancer. Sucralose has been shown to spike your insulin more than sugar and change how your body responds to carbohydrates, while aspartame is related to health effects ranging from mild problems such as headaches, dizziness, digestive symptoms, and changes in mood, to more serious health issues such as Alzheimer's disease, birth defects, diabetes, Gulf War syndrome, attention deficit disorders, Parkinson's disease, lupus, multiple sclerosis, and seizures. Studies leading to FDA approval have recently ruled out cancer risk for the most part. However, those studies were done using far smaller amounts of diet soda than the 24 ounces a day consumed by many people who drink this product. This means we really don't know what effect large amounts of these chemicals will have over many years. Additionally, there have been no long-term studies of the effects of these substitutes as they are fairly new to the market. The same thing happened with tobacco; it took years to track the dangerous effects of smoking cigarettes.

So, before crowding out sugar from your diet, do yourself a favor and check your food labels at home and throw out everything that has on its label:

- Aspartame

- Acesulfame Potassium (K)

- Saccharin or sucralose

- NutraSweet®

- Splenda®

And avoid products that are labeled 'low-calorie', 'diet', 'sugar-free', or 'no sugar added' since they all likely contain sugar additives.

SODA

Did you know that drinking a single 330ml can of soda each day translates to more than 1lb of weight gain every month? Agh! I know!

This is a topic dear to a lot of people: soda. Soda is one of the most consumed beverages in the United States, second only to water. There are really **no nutritional benefits** in soft drinks. They mostly consist of filtered water, sugar, and sometime colorants or additives for flavor.

Many regular soda drinkers know that soda is bad for their health, yet the average American drinks about 57 gallons of soft drinks each year. Have you ever stopped and wondered why we can't stop consuming it? Let's take a look at what happens to your body when you chug a soft drink:

As soon as soda is swallowed, the pancreas responds to the sugar by beginning to create insulin (a hormone the body uses to move sugar from food or drink into the bloodstream and transform into energy). Within just 20 minutes, **blood-sugar levels spike** and the liver responds to the insulin by turning sugar into fat for storage.

Within 45 minutes, the caffeine in soda is fully absorbed, raising your blood pressure. This creates a feeling of excitement, similar to that of amphetamines, and the body begins to produce more of the chemical in your brain that affects your emotions, movements, and your sensations of pleasure. When these levels rise significantly, it stimulates the pleasure centers of the brain and makes you crave more. The mechanism is exactly the same with drugs like cocaine. And this is when and how you get addicted.

Besides the addiction problem, soda makes you gain weight and dissolves bone mass due to the citric acid contained in it. Studies have also found that soda messes with blood pressure, increases the risk of heart disease, and can cause some serious reproductive issues. And it doesn't end there... Did you know that for every can of soda you drink per day, your risk of obesity increases by 60 percent[xvii]?!

WHAT ABOUT DIET SODA?

There has been a long-standing diet soda debate over whether it's healthier than regular soda or not. In the conventional nutritional world, which is primarily concerned with counting calories, diet drinks are encouraged as the preferred zero-calorie option. On the other hand, research has correlated a 66% increase risk of diabetes with consuming just 20 ounces of diet soda per week!

As if that isn't enough, all diet drinks contain sugar substitutes and artificial sugars that, as mentioned before, do more harm than good to your health. Some of the risks related to these are cancers, behavioral disorders, thyroid issues, and much more.

In the Multi-Ethnic Study of Atherosclerosis (MESA), daily consumption of diet drinks was associated with a 36% greater risk for metabolic syndrome and a 67% increased risk for Type II diabetes. Aren't these the diseases that artificial sweeteners are supposed to help prevent in the first place?

So, what should you do? Ditching soda is one of the easiest changes you can make to significantly improve your health. There are many alternatives to soda that can be just as satisfying. Here are my favorite go-to drinks:

Kombucha: Kombucha is a fermented tea that typically includes a mixture of yeast, good bacteria, a natural sweetener, and black tea. It's an antioxidant-rich drink with organic acids, enzymes, probiotics, and B vitamins full of benefits. It's fizzy like soda, but very low in sugar at just 2 grams per 8-ounce serving versus 27 grams for soda. IMPORTANT TIP: Make sure your kombucha is raw. Pasteurized kombucha is high in sugar and has very few of the health benefits compared with its raw counterpart because the good bacteria have been destroyed.

Water with fruit: Adding fruit to a pitcher of ice-cold water can make for a refreshing and flavorful drink. If you crave the bubbles, try adding some fruit juice to your seltzer water and sweeten it with raw honey.

Coconut water: I am personally not a fan of coconut water as I find it too sweet for my taste, but I have recommended it to some of my clients in the past to help in transitioning from sodas. Coconut water has many health benefits, including a lot of potassium and natural minerals. Something to note, though: coconut water contains natural sugar (although less than soda per ml) and the amount of sugar contained in a typical bottle can be over two teaspoons. It is wise to watch the amount consumed and perhaps only add a splash of it to your regular water for taste, especially if you are used to consuming multiple sodas per day.

Sparkling water: If what you love about soda is the carbonation, try sparkling water. You can enjoy it with added flavors like cucumber, mint, or berries, or squeeze some fruit into it.

Tea: There are so many different brands and flavors to enjoy. It's all about finding the one that works best for you. You can also chill the tea or add it to cold sparkling water with a little honey to make a fresh fizzy drink.

The bottom line is, try to remember as a general guideline that your best bet for hydrating yourself, as always, is water.

TRY: SUGAR-FREE WEEK

Now that you understand why it is important for you to limit your sugar intake, especially artificial sweeteners, it's time to become a sugar detective. This week, you'll be focusing your attention on scanning the labels of your food and looking for any added artificial and processed sugars. So, get ready!

SWEET TRANSITION

I'll be the first to admit that cutting sugar from your diet is no easy task. What you'll experience when you ditch the sweet stuff will depend on how much sugar you have been consuming and for how long. If you ingest a lot of sugar or you have consumed sugar for a long period of time (as in years), be aware that you could show addict-like withdrawal symptoms, including: dizziness, confusion, anxiety, headaches, restlessness, fatigue, mood swings, and even depression. Other symptoms experienced by people who have detoxed from sugar include:

- Muscle aches and pains
- Nausea
- Chills or sweats
- Insomnia
- Strange dreams
- Boredom
- Gas and bloating

But don't get discouraged. Here are a few tricks to help calm the symptoms:

Eat every two to three hours for the first few days of your transition: Try to eat some protein, animal or vegan, along with a vegetable; for example, hummus with carrots. This will help prevent hypoglycemia and stabilize your blood sugar. Even after your system has adjusted, it is wise to eat four to six small meals a day. Eating more frequently has been shown to normalize cholesterol levels and will also help your adrenal glands better regulate cortisol levels.

Eat sweet and root vegetables: Sweet vegetables like beets, sweet potatoes, and onions are great replacements for refined sugar. If you're really craving sugar, a beet salad, or roasted, sweet root vegetables could be just what you need to get your fix.

Get more exercise: Breaking a sweat helps take your mind off sugar and balance out your body, bringing it to a more alkaline state. By sweating out extra salt, your sugar craving is greatly reduced. Try to start your day off with a workout. If you do this, then you are more likely to make healthier choices when it comes to your food intake all day long.

Cut out processed food: If you haven't already, try to avoid processed food. Almost all processed foods are packed full of secret sugars that fuel your addiction. Just read the label of that bread, cereal, milk, or yogurt in your kitchen! When you're trying to quit sugar, it's best to go back to basics and eat only fresh foods.

Find a buddy: As with any health and wellness goal, achieving a sugar-free lifestyle is always much easier when you have a partner. Set up a daily text message exchange with this person so you can offer words of support and encouragement when one of you is feeling tempted by the donuts in the break room at work. You might even consider swapping healthy recipes or making time to go to the gym together.

Take an L-glutamine supplement (1000-2000mg) every day: Glutamine often relieves sugar cravings as the brain uses it for fuel.

Distract yourself, go for a walk, or take a break to do some breathing exercises: Find a quiet spot, get comfortable and sit for a few minutes and focus on your breath. Cravings usually last for 10 to 20 minutes maximum. If you can distract yourself with something else, it often passes.

Avoid extreme hunger: Extreme hunger can lead to poor decision-making. Plan your meals and snacks.

Keep sugary foods out of your house: Stock your cupboards with healthy foods that will keep you satisfied throughout the day.

Manage stress: If you have stress, look into relaxation techniques such as meditation, yoga, or massage.

Ditch all artificial sweeteners too: As explained before, using artificial sweeteners is not good for your health and may increase your sugar cravings. I strongly recommend *avoiding all artificial sweeteners* and reading food labels to make sure you're not inadvertently consuming them. They're added to some 6,000 different beverages, snacks, and food products, so you really need to pay attention to the labels. Unfortunately, just like sugar, artificial sweeteners can cause you to become addicted.

Now, it would be pretty hard and rather extreme to spend the rest of your life avoiding sugar till the end. By now, you know I'm all about balance. So, the question is: How do you find balance between your sweet tooth or the desire to sweeten certain foods and drinks, and doing so in a healthy way?

BEST SUGAR ALTERNATIVES

What to use to sweeten your food is a popular subject, given that it's becoming widely known that refined sugar is one of the worst foods you can eat. When choosing an alternative to sugar, you have to be cautious because most of the options out there may actually be worse for you than real sugar, including artificial sweeteners as we saw before.

Natural sweeteners are always preferable to refined sugar and high fructose corn syrup, because they have less of a negative impact on your body. Transitioning to sweeteners like *raw unfiltered honey, raw cane sugar, agave nectar, date sugar, or coconut sugar* can ease the daily stress that a sweet diet can create in the body.

Let's take a close look at the best sugar alternatives:

Raw unfiltered honey: Unheated and unfiltered honey is my favorite sweetener of all. It retains its natural enzymes, antioxidants, minerals, and vitamins and research shows it has antimicrobial properties. Just be sure to pick raw unfiltered wildflower honey.

Stevia: Found in Central and South America, this herb is up to 200 times sweeter than sugar but since it's not metabolized it won't cause a jump in your blood sugar. *Cons:* Stevia might not be for everyone because of its bitter, licorice-like aftertaste. If stevia won't cut it for you, try Truvia or SweetLeaf, which use only the sweetest parts of the plant in their products.

Coconut sugar: Made from the boiled, dehydrated sap of the coconut palm, coconut sugar has a lower GI (glycemic index) than table sugar. *Cons:* Just like other sweeteners, it still contains lots of sugar, so use it sparingly.

Molasses: Blackstrap molasses is the thick liquid produced during cane sugar processing after the maximum amount of sugar crystals are removed. The taste is usually rich, subtly smoky, and bittersweet. It's higher in vitamins and minerals than most sweeteners and has a lower GI than table sugar. *Cons:* Some people find it slightly bitter, so it may be more difficult to substitute for sugar in some cases.

Date sugar: Date sugar is simply powdered dried dates. It is a bit less sweet than other natural sweeteners but retains some nutrients from whole dates such as small amounts of fiber, calcium, potassium, and magnesium. Cons: It doesn't dissolve in drinks, so it's best sprinkled on foods.

Maple syrup: Real maple syrup is made by boiling the sap extracted from maple trees, which evaporates the water content and transforms into a concentrated, sweet syrup. *Cons:* Unfortunately, the most commonly used kind that graces many diners and pantries here in the US is made from high fructose corn syrup and caramel coloring. If you're going to buy maple syrup, then make sure to get actual maple syrup, not just maple-*flavored* syrup. Look for the wording 'Grade A' on the label. And please do not confuse maple syrup with 'pancake syrup' as they are two completely different things. Regardless, I prefer to steer clear of maple syrup except on rare occasions as, even in its purest form, it has a high sugar content.

Keep in mind that **replacing refined sugar** with pure, quality natural sugar is likely to yield a net health benefit but *adding* it to your diet will just make things worse. So, if you don't regularly add sugar to your food and drink, or you don't have a sweet tooth, this is not the time to start.

BOTTOM LINE: It's all about balance. Sugar-containing foods in their natural form, such as whole fruit, for example, tend to be highly nutritious — nutrient-dense, high in fiber, low in glycemic load. On the other hand, refined, concentrated sugar consumed in large amounts rapidly increases blood glucose and insulin levels, increases triglycerides, inflammatory mediators, and oxygen radicals, and with them, the risk of diabetes, cardiovascular disease, and other chronic illnesses.

When eliminating sugar, you may notice an increase in taste, more constant energy levels, and fewer mid-afternoon crashes, which will leave you feeling good all day long.

After this week off sugar, you may start feeling improvements in your energy levels and mood, but some people may still be stuck with withdrawal symptoms. Be gentle with yourself. Ditching sugar is not an easy task and you may fail a couple of times before you succeed. Let go of the guilt and keep trying. It takes many failures to change a habit, especially with this kind of addiction. Nourish your body with healthy foods, develop a true compassion toward yourself, and be patient.

No matter what, just try to stick with it. You are strong. I know you can do this!

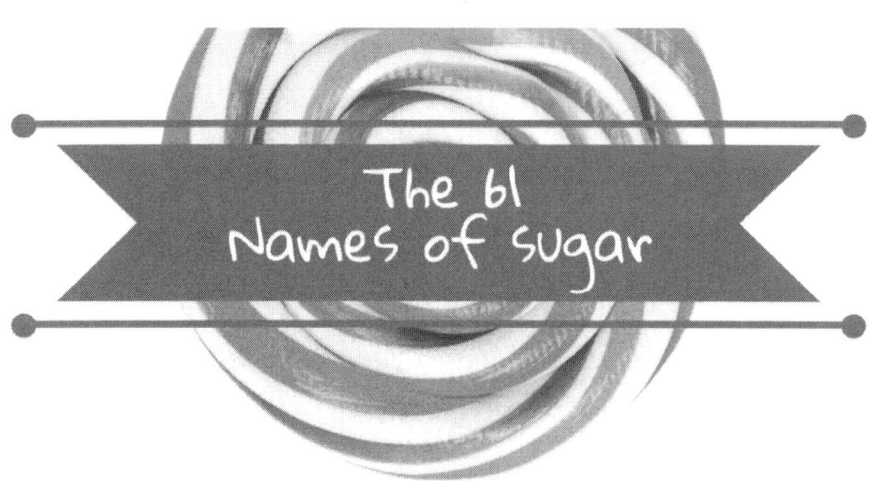

The 61 Names of Sugar

Agave nectar

Barbados sugar

Barley malt

Barley malt syrup

Beet sugar

Brown sugar

Buttered syrup

Cane juice

Cane juice crystals

Cane sugar

Caramel

Carob syrup

Castor sugar

Coconut palm sugar

Coconut sugar

Confectioner's sugar

Corn sweetener

Corn syrup

Corn syrup solids

Date sugar

Dehydrated cane juice

Demerara sugar

Dextrin

DextroseEvaporated cane juice

Free-flowing brown sugars

Fructose

Fruit juice

Fruit juice concentrate

Glucose

Glucose solids

Golden sugar

Golden syrup

Grape sugar

HFCS (high-fructose corn syrup)

Honey

Icing sugar

Invert sugar

Malt syrup

Maltodextrin

Maltol

Maltose

Mannose

Maple syrup

Molasses

Muscovado

Palm sugar

Panocha

Powdered sugar

Raw sugar

Refiner's syrup

Rice syrup

Saccharose

Sorghum syrup

Sucrose

Sugar (granulated)

Sweet sorghum

Syrup

Treacle

Turbinado sugar

Yellow sugar

CHECK-IN QUESTIONS

How were your energy levels on a scale of 1 to 10?

Did you feel fatigued or sluggish?

Can you think clearly?

Did you feel tired?

Did you feel bloated?

Did you have headaches? (If yes, how many?)

Did you go to the bathroom regularly?

Is your skin clear?

Did you have cravings?

Did you binge?

Did you eat or snack compulsively or mindlessly?

Is your sleep regular?

Did you have trouble concentrating or brain fog?

Did you suffer with mood swings?

Did you ever feel anxious, fearful, or nervous?

Did you feel physically weak?

Did you get sick?

Did you have bad breath?

Did you have heartburn?

Did you have stomach or intestinal pain?

Did you experience ringing in your ears?

Did you feel the need to urinate urgently or frequently?

Did you have pain or aches in your muscles and joints?

Did you feel stiff or limited in your movements?

"Gluten free, vegan, fat-free… Gosh, I love this champagne diet."

WEEK 6

SHOULD YOU BE GLUTEN-FREE?

Gluten is currently considered the greatest of evils in our popular nutrition world, like carbs were in the 90s and fat was in the 80s. Going gluten-free seems to be the latest dietary sensation with 63% of Americans believing that following a gluten-free diet will improve their physical and mental health, according to a 2014 Consumer Reports[xviii] survey. Indeed, over 41% of Americans are actively trying to avoid gluten.

But are there any real benefits in being gluten-free, or is this just a new trend?

Unfortunately, a whole lot of what's 'common knowledge' on gluten today is a result of popularity, smart marketing, and internet gossip. So, should you eat gluten or not? Before we answer this question, we need to clarify the confusion and start from the very beginning. This chapter explains what gluten is, and how and why it can affect your health.

Let's get to it.

WHAT IS GLUTEN?

Gluten is a protein molecule principally found in wheat, rye, and barley, and their various forms (durum, bulgur, emmer, spelt, farina, farro, kamut, khorasan, wheat, triticale, and einkorn). This protein is best known for giving baked goods their doughy, elastic structure. However, many foods contain gluten for other purposes, including as a thickening agent or flavor enhancer.

The main sources of gluten are:

Wheat, as commonly found in:

- Breads
- Baked goods
- Soups
- Pasta
- Cereals
- Sauces
- Salad dressings
- Roux

Barley, as commonly found in:

- Malt
- Food coloring
- Soups
- Malt vinegar
- Beer

Rye, as commonly found in:

- Rye bread, such as pumpernickel
- Rye beer
- Cereals

Triticale: This is a new hybrid cereal, created by crossbreeding wheat and rye. The goal of this genetically engineered grain is to have a similar growing quality as wheat, while being tolerant to a variety of growing conditions like rye.

Triticale can potentially be found in:

- Breads

- Pasta

- Cereals

WHEN GLUTEN WENT 'BAD'

In the late 60s, wheat was crossbred, hybridized, and re-engineered to increase the yield of certain grains and give more elasticity to baked goods like bread, etc. This has produced 40,000 different varieties of wheat that do not exist in nature. Because of this action, the gluten molecule has changed from the cellular equivalent of a tennis ball to the size of volleyball!

Now, it's not hard to understand that the larger the protein molecule, the more challenging it is for your digestive system to break it down fully, which is why there has been a rise in gluten intolerance.

THE SCOOP ON LEAKY GUT

The truth is that the real issue is not with gluten but with gliadin, which has changed tremendously as a result of the re-engineered version of wheat. So, how does gliadin help us unravel the gluten mystery?

Gliadin is a protein found in wheat gluten and is essential for giving bread and baked products the ability to rise properly during baking. Because of the re-engineering, these proteins can now affect our bodies in many different ways. Here are some of the important points that we know about gliadin:

- Most gluten sensitivity is really a gliadin sensitivity.

- Gliadin is degraded to a collection of polypeptides called *exorphins* in the gastrointestinal tract. Exorphins cross the blood-brain barrier and bind (tie tightly) to opiate receptors to induce appetite, as well as behavioral changes (such as behavioral outbursts and inattention) in children with ADHD and autism, hearing voices and social detachment in schizophrenics, and the mania of bipolar illness.

- Gliadin acts as an opiate, causing addiction to wheat and a stimulation of the appetite for carbohydrates.

- Gliadin is capable of binding to nervous system tissue and may contribute to immune-mediated neurological impairment, such as cerebellar ataxia (which can prevent you from walking properly, balance while sitting, co-ordinate arms, hands, legs, eye movements, and speech) and very bad headaches.

- Gliadin weakens the tight junctions that seal the lining of the gut by opening up gaps in the intestinal walls, allowing toxins and undigested food to enter the bloodstream. This is what is known as 'leaky gut', which you might have heard about. This is what gets us into trouble.

Scientists have discovered that the tight junctions between the cells in the gut lining must be strong, or else you can incur countless diseases and disorders, like celiac disease, multiple sclerosis, Type I diabetes, cancer, allergies, and more.

A healthy gut, on the other hand, is completely sealed and will only allow nutrients and small molecules to pass through. Strong tight junctions will aid in nutrient absorption, fight off infection, and balance the inner ecosystem.

WHAT ABOUT CELIAC DISEASE?

Celiac disease (CD) AKA gluten intolerance is not an allergy, but an autoimmune condition in your gut. In brief, it works like this for people with celiac disease: When gluten reaches their gut, the immune system mistakenly believes the gluten is a foreign invader (like a bacteria). This causes the immune system to mount an **attack on the molecule of gluten** and intestine wall, irritating the gut and flattening the microvilli along the small intestine wall. Without these microvilli, the body cannot absorb nutrients from their food, which leads them to experience symptoms of malabsorption.

The most common symptoms are digestive discomfort, anemia, chronic fatigue, depression, deficiencies, neurological disorders, nausea, skin rashes, and a difficulty in gaining weight. Celiac disease often has few to no symptoms, which is why it is estimated that only 30% of people with the disease are diagnosed. The remaining 60% are undiagnosed or misdiagnosed with other conditions. Other signs or common symptoms of possible celiac disease are:

- Iron-deficiency anemia

- Joint pain and stiffness

- Bone pain

- Bone loss or osteoporosis

- Depression or anxiety

- Canker sores inside the mouth

- Itchy skin rash (dermatitis herpetiformis)

- Fatigue

- Seizures or migraines

- Numbness and tingling in the hands and feet

- Tooth discoloration or loss of enamel

- Pale sores inside the mouth

- Irregular menstrual periods

- Infertility and miscarriage

- Weight loss

- Vomiting

- Abdominal bloating

- Abdominal pain

- Persistent diarrhea or constipation

- Pale, fatty, foul-smelling stools

Some conditions associated with celiac disease also include:

- Lupus

- Rheumatoid arthritis

- Type 1 diabetes

- Thyroid disease

- Autoimmune liver disease

- Addison's disease

- Sjogren's syndrome

- Down syndrome

- Turner syndrome

- Lactose intolerance

- Intestinal cancer

- Intestinal lymphoma

If you suffer from any of the above symptoms, I highly recommend you go and get tested for celiac disease. There are two main ways to find out if you have celiac disease:

Blood tests: There are several blood tests that screen for antibodies. The most common one is called the tTG-IgA test. If this is positive, a tissue biopsy is usually recommended to confirm the results.

Biopsy from small intestine: A health professional takes a small tissue sample from the small intestine, which is analyzed for damage.

If you test negative to celiac disease, but still react badly to gluten, it's likely you suffer with non-celiac gluten sensitivity (NCGS). The symptoms are similar to those with CD, but antibodies to gluten are not produced nor is there intestinal damage (two hallmarks of celiac disease).

Some of the most common symptoms of NCGS are: diagnosis of an autoimmune disease, brain fog, mood issues (such as depression, anxiety, and ADHD-like behavior), abdominal pain, bloating, diarrhea, constipation, headaches, dizziness, inflammation, fibromyalgia, bone or joint pain, keratosis pilaris (also known as 'chicken skin') on the backs of arms, and chronic fatigue.

NCGS is still a matter of debate. Indirect evidence suggests that NCGS is more common than CD[xix], although a recently published study[xx] in the journal *Digestion* found that 86% of individuals who **believed** they were gluten-sensitive could actually tolerate it. NCGS may be transient and could be as a result of damaged gut flora (AKA dysbiosis), which is on the rise in our society for a number of reasons: too much sugar, alcohol, antibiotics, environmental toxins, and other allergens recently introduced to our foods (like GMOs). All of these contribute to imbalanced intestinal flora, which can lead to gluten-sensitivity.

TRY: GLUTEN-FREE WEEK

So, should you eat gluten or not? This question is a hot topic and the bottom line is you must avoid gluten if you are celiac, although a recent survey suggests celiac disease only affects 1% of the population. This means **you can eat gluten** but doing so on a daily basis and not taking any supplement to strengthen your stomach lining is not ideal.

If after reading this chapter you think you may have celiac disease, you should consult with your doctor and get tested before trying a gluten-free diet. If you tested negative to CD but want to find out if you react badly to gluten, you may want to try to eliminate gluten from your diet for two to three weeks and then to reintroduce it to see if your symptoms return.

In order to get accurate results from this testing method, you must eliminate 100% of the gluten in your diet. And by 100%, I mean 100%. The 80/20 rule or "I don't eat gluten at home, just when I go out" attitude won't work, as you send yourself back to the beginning every time you put gluten in your stomach.

Now, I know eliminating gluten can be confusing and overwhelming, so below is a chart of what you can and can't eat during the following weeks:

OFF-LIMITS INGREDIENTS:

- Barley
- Bulgur

- Couscous
- Cracked wheat

- Durum and durum flour

- Einkorn

- Emmer

- Farina

- Farro

- Fu (common in Asian foods)

- Gliadin

- Graham flour

- Kamut

- Malt, malt flavoring, and malt vinegar

(usually made from barley)

- Matzo

- Rye

- Semolina

- Spelt

- Triticale (a cross between wheat and rye)

- Wheat

- Wheat starch

- Wheat bran

- Wheat germ

OFF- LIMITS FOODS:

- Beer

- Breads

- Cakes and pies

- Candy

- Cereals

- Cookies and crackers

- Croutons

- Dairy (unless from grass fed animals)

- French fries

- Gravy

- Imitation meat or seafood

- Matzo

- Pastas

- Processed luncheon meats

- Sauces

- Seasoned rice mixes

- Seasoned snack foods, such as potato and tortilla chips

- Self-basting poultry

- Soups and soup bases

- Vegetables in sauce

Gluten may also show up as ingredients in barley malt, chicken broth, malt vinegar, some salad dressings, veggie burgers (if not specified gluten-free), and soy sauce. The protein may even hide in many common seasonings and spice mixes.

Now, I know that eliminating all of the above can be quite a challenge, so if you really can't live without some of the foods mentioned above, you can opt for their gluten-free version.

BE AWARE: Gluten free foods aren't automatically better for you. Plenty of them can make you gain unwanted weight. In fact, it's not uncommon to gain up to 20lbs within the first year of a gluten-free diet. The main reason is that most gluten-free alternatives available nowadays on the market are highly processed and loaded with fat, sugar, and sodium to replace gluten and maintain a good taste or consistency. Be sure to scan the ingredient labels before replacing your dear bread, cookies, and cereals, or you might end up feeling worse and gaining weight instead of detoxing your body.

If you pay close attention, all the off-limits foods mentioned above are processed foods. It may seem daunting at first, but thankfully, there are plenty of foods that are naturally gluten-free. Please feel free to eat any of the below:

- Fruit
- Vegetables
- Beans
- Seeds
- Legumes
- Nuts
- Potatoes

- Eggs
- Dairy products
- Corn
- Rice
- Fish
- Lean beef
- Chicken

Other grains and foods that are also gluten-free:

- Amaranth
- Arrowroot
- Buckwheat
- Cassava
- Corn and cornmeal (please buy organic)
- Flax
- Gluten-free flours (rice, soy, corn, potato, bean)

- Millet
- Quinoa
- Rice
- Sorghum
- Soy
- Tapioca
- Teff

Seek out an integrative practitioner like myself to help guide you through the process and address your doubts, concerns, or challenges.

BOTTOM LINE: You should not go on a gluten-free diet to try to lose weight. Gluten is not your enemy. Unless you have tested positive for celiac disease or other autoimmune conditions, consuming gluten in moderation (such as two to three times a week, not on a daily basis) should not affect your health. Just like with everything else, always try to source the highest quality possible of gluten-containing foods and choose sprouted grains, flour, and breads as they are easier to digest.

As a side note, by reducing gluten-containing products, you will help yourself reduce many of the processed foods and carbohydrates that may well be contributing to the obesity epidemic. Eating a meal that is free of processed ingredients, and full of tasty, hearty vegetables and proteins instead, is going to be much healthier for you anyway.

Just keep in mind to always trust your intuition. If you think you react negatively to gluten, you should consult your doctor and get tested for celiac disease. When that's ruled out, a gluten-free diet may help determine if you're actually gluten-intolerant or if you have a leaky gut, which are both reversible. See the next chapter for more detail.

If your symptoms don't improve on a gluten-free diet, and don't get worse when you reintroduce gluten, then the culprit is probably something else.

CHECK-IN QUESTIONS

How were your energy levels on a scale of 1 to 10?

Did you feel fatigued or sluggish?

Can you think clearly?

Did you feel tired?

Did you feel bloated?

Did you have headaches? (If yes, how many?)

Did you go to the bathroom regularly?

Is your skin clear?

Did you have cravings?

Did you binge?

Did you eat or snack compulsively or mindlessly?

Is your sleep regular?

Did you have trouble concentrating or brain fog?

Did you suffer with mood swings?

Did you ever feel anxious, fearful, or nervous?

Did you feel physically weak?

Did you get sick?

Did you have bad breath?

Did you have heartburn?

Did you have stomach or intestinal pain?

Did you experience ringing in your ears?

Did you feel the need to urinate urgently or frequently?

Did you have pain or aches in your muscles and joints?

Did you feel stiff or limited in your movements?

*"Siri: take me
to this kitchen
where abs are made."*

WEEK 7

FLAT STOMACH, MORE ENERGY

Yes, believe it or not, the two do go hand in hand.

By now you've likely heard of the gut microbiome and maybe you're even aware of some of the myriad benefits mighty microbes can have on your health. But did you know that a thriving gut is one of the most important keys to a balanced and fulfilled life? In fact, a healthy gut can help with:

- Sharpening your focus
- Giving you a natural energy boost
- Finding and maintaining your ideal weight
- Supporting your immune system
- Boosting your mood
- Giving you a glowing complexion
- Having a flat stomach

The issue is that, in our current society, we give our digestive systems plenty of work to do. As explained at the beginning of this book, our evolution from the hunter-gatherer diet to convenient and fast food has overwhelmed our metabolism and gastrointestinal (GI) tract, all in favor of inflammation.

Our modern diet offers too much sugar and carbs, high levels of wheat, dairy, and other common allergens, with not enough fatty acids, which are vital to fight off inflammation.

This week we will focus our attention on fighting off the inflammation in our bodies, specifically by restoring our gut health.

Why are we going to address our gut health? Well, two-thirds of the body's defenses reside in the GI tract, as it is the apparatus that was designed by nature to eliminate viruses and bacteria in your food before they infect your body. Most inflammatory diseases start in the gut with an autoimmune reaction, which progresses into systemic inflammation.

Intestinal bloating, brain fog, frequent bouts of diarrhea or constipation, gas and pain, heartburn, and acid reflux are all early signs of an inflamed digestive tract. Systemic or chronic inflammation has a domino effect that can seriously undermine your health as your body cannot properly eliminate toxins or accomplish its regular vital functions.

For all the symptoms of inflammation, refresh your memory by referring back to Week 1.

Addressing the friendly flora that resides in your gut can put you on the fast track to your most productive, accomplished, and satisfied life ever!

TRY: HEAL YOUR GUT WEEK

If you follow this chapter's recommendations, you may also help reverse some food intolerances. If you ruled out gluten last week, I suggest you keep it out of your diet during this upcoming week too.

To reduce inflammation and heal your gut, you have different options. If you have a chronic condition, or severe symptoms of inflammation, I encourage you to work with an integrative healthcare practitioner or functional medicine provider to create a plan that suits your unique needs.

Below is my favorite protocol, which you can implement on your own.

1. Remove

The goal is to get rid of inflammatory foods, infections, and gastric irritants. Inflammatory foods are **gluten, dairy, corn, soy, and sugar**. In addition, **caffeine and alcohol** need to be removed in this first phase as they add stress to the body, prevent proper nutrient absorption, and can feed candida. Over time, coffee and alcohol may be consumed in small quantities, but not on a daily basis.

Also avoid:

Processed oils: Soybean, sunflower, corn, canola, cottonseed, safflower and vegetable oil, corn, soybean, and other oils that are usually overheated or processed to a degree that makes the oil difficult to digest.

Processed or treated meats: Avoid deli or lunch meat, as the chemicals used for treatment can cause inflammation and irritate the intestinal lining. Meat treated with antibiotics can create immune-suppressing activity in your body.

Artificial sweeteners: Artificial sweeteners are synthetic, can cause stress and inflammation in the gut, and may be derived from ingredients your body is allergic to.

Additives and packaged foods: As we saw in the processed food chapter in Week 3, these all cause inflammation.

Flavorings: Any flavorings, artificial or natural, come from unknown sources that may irritate the gut.

The following are gray-area foods, as not everyone can properly digest them.

Legumes, nuts, and grains: Quinoa too, despite its growing popularity as a healthy grain, can actually be hard to digest for many people. If you consume nuts, legumes, or grains because you think you are doing your body a favor, try to pay attention to how you feel afterwards. If you get bloated, extremely tired, have diarrhea or constipation after you eat any of these, try to avoid them.

Nightshades: While these vegetables all have beneficial nutrients, they are considered toxic because of a natural pesticide in them – glycol-alkaloids — which is believed to harm red blood cells. In general, it's best to limit these, but people with autoimmune diseases should consider avoiding nightshades completely.

Here is a complete list of edible nightshades:

- Bell peppers (a.k.a. sweet peppers)
- Bush tomato
- Cape gooseberry (do not confuse with regular cherries)
- Cocona
- Eggplant
- Goji berries (a.k.a. wolfberry)
- Garden huckleberry (do not confuse with regular huckleberries)
- Kutjera

- Hot peppers (chili peppers, jalapenos, habaneros, chili-based spices, red pepper, cayenne)

- Naranjillas

- Paprika

- Pepinos

- Pimentos

- Potatoes (but not sweet potatoes)

- Tomatillos

- Tomatoes

- Tamarillos

SIDE NOTE: Consult with your physician for a comprehensive exam to determine the levels of good bacteria as well as any infections present in your blood or stool. Removing the infections may require treatment with herbs, anti-parasite medication, anti-fungal medication, or even antibiotics.

2. Replenish

Add back into your gut the essential ingredients for proper digestion and absorption that may have been depleted by diet, drugs (such as antacid medications), diseases, or aging. It has been found that beneficial microflora will release anti-inflammatory messages and dampen the inflammatory response. Take a good probiotic before going to bed (80-100 billion units), consider using digestive enzymes like papaya, and take liquid chloroxygen drops in your water once a day.

3. Repair

Providing the nutrients necessary to help the gut repair itself is essential. The surface area of your gut is lined with a type of cell that regenerates every 2 to 3 weeks! Thanks to this quick turnaround, those without chronic gut problems can heal their gut in as little as 2 to 12 weeks. But if you have autoimmune-inflammation issues or a fully damaged gut it can take between 12 and 24 months to completely heal and notice sustainable changes. So, depending on your current situation, I suggest you try the recommendation below for a month at first. If you feel a difference, stick with it for a further 3 to 6 months:

L-glutamine: Glutamine is considered the most important nutrient for healing 'leaky gut syndrome'. This is one of my favorite supplements, an amino acid that helps to rejuvenate the gut wall lining. But unlike many of the other amino acids, it is unique, because it is the primary fuel used by the cells in your gut lining and your cells can actually absorb it directly! What superstars!

One of the main issues in taking L-glutamine is the conflicting dosage information that is available. The recommended dose on the packaging is usually not enough to repair the gut, but only enough to maintain it. If you're trying to *heal* your gut, you may have to follow a more drastic protocol for a few days (Charles Poliquin being the most famous one). To me, his approach was a little too aggressive, so when I did some research, I made my own program, which goes as follows:

STEP1: CALCULATE IDEAL DOSE

After some research, I found a good rule of thumb that helps ensure you get enough L-glutamine each day, which is 0.5g of L-glutamine per kilo of body weight.

(60kg body weight) x (0.5g L-glutamine) = 30g of L-glutamine per day

STEP 2: WORK YOUR WAY UP

I recommend starting with a lower dose and slowly work your way up to a larger dose to make sure that your body tolerates the supplement well. Start with 5g and increase it every three days.

STEP 3: MEGADOSE

Sit on your ideal dose for a minimum of five days and see how you do with it. If your body responds well, you can continue with this dose for a month or two, depending on how your symptoms go.

STEP 4: TAPER OFF

Taper off to a smaller long-term dose of 5 to 10mg per day.

Aloe vera: All-time superstar! I start every day with a warm glass of water with aloe vera juice (or apple cider vinegar. I alternate them). Aloe is highly detoxifying, soothes the stomach, helps with digestion and nutrient absorption, allows the gut tissue to heal and protects it from further injury or infiltration by bacteria.

Omega-3s: They are also essential for managing inflammation, blood clotting, and brain development. International guidelines suggest we should consume 250 milligrams of omega-3 a day (and up to 500 mg).

Gold standard organic sulfur: Sulfur makes up vital amino acids used to create protein for cells and tissues, hormones, enzymes, and antibodies. The body uses up its store daily so it must be continually replenished for optimal health and nutrition. That's why I recommend you add it to your daily practice. Having enough sulfur also helps your body remove toxins. To help repair your gut, take one teaspoon, three times daily for two weeks and then continue twice a day for the following two weeks. You can find it for sale on Amazon.

Just be sure to search the right term: 'gold standard organic sulfur'.

BOTTOM LINE: A healthy digestive tract is key for overall heath. Consuming fiber and nutrient-rich foods and eliminating or limiting inflammatory foods are two great starting points to improve your gut health. Remember to repair the damage that has been done so far. The repair phase can last anywhere between two weeks and 12 to 24 months if you suffer with any autoimmune disease. **Please always remember to speak to your doctor before starting any sort of supplement.**

CHECK-IN QUESTIONS

How were your energy levels on a scale of 1 to 10?

Did you feel fatigued or sluggish?

Can you think clearly?

Did you feel tired?

Did you feel bloated?

Did you have headaches? (If yes, how many?)

Did you go to the bathroom regularly?

Is your skin clear?

Did you have cravings?

Did you binge?

Did you eat or snack compulsively or mindlessly?

Is your sleep regular?

Did you have trouble concentrating or brain fog?

Did you suffer with mood swings?

Did you ever feel anxious, fearful, or nervous?

Did you feel physically weak?

Did you get sick?

Did you have bad breath?

Did you have heartburn?

Did you have stomach or intestinal pain?

Did you experience ringing in your ears?

Did you feel the need to urinate urgently or frequently?

Did you have pain or aches in your muscles and joints?

Did you feel stiff or limited in your movements?

"I just found out I have IBES…
Irritable Because of
Everything Syndrome."

WEEK 8

IBS and FODMAP

By now, you should be entering your third week without gluten. How are you feeling? Do you feel more alert? Do you have more energy? Are you still bloated?

Millions of people live with undiagnosed bouts of bloating, constipation, and diarrhea and consider it normal. In fact, it has been estimated that irritable bowel syndrome alone affects one in every five Americans and two every ten people in the UK. Pretty crazy, no? IBS can come with debilitating stomach pain, diarrhea, or constipation, and can have a serious impact on the sufferer's quality of life but can go beyond bathroom problems. Because of the gut-brain connection, as many as 90% of people with IBS also have psychiatric disorders, including panic disorders, generalized anxiety disorders, and major depression.

So, what can you do to improve IBS symptoms, if going gluten-free did not solve your issues? There is a new dietary approach that has recently become more popular, a strategy that I have seen work well for many of my clients, also known as the low FODMAP diet.

WHAT ARE FODMAPs?

FODMAP stands for Fermentable Oligosaccharides, Disaccharides, Monosaccharides, and Polyols. In short, fermentable sugars. These short-chain carbohydrates are not completely absorbed in your intestine and can be easily fermented by gut bacteria. The fermentation and osmosis caused by these undigested sugars are a cause of the major IBS symptoms such as gas, pain, and diarrhea. Many common foods are high in FODMAPs and can potentially contribute to IBS symptoms, even if they are considered 'healthy' foods by most standards.

WHAT CAUSES IBS AND FODMAP INTOLERANCE?

Although the exact causes of IBS are, as yet, unknown, there are a few possible explanations that have been explored in clinical studies. In some cases, researchers notice that small intestinal bacterial overgrowth contributes to the development of IBS symptoms and FODMAP intolerance. In other cases, they discovered certain people may lack adequate enzymes to break down FODMAP foods before they reach the colon, which contributes to their fermentation and further allows the proliferation of uncontrolled gut bacteria.

Emotional and physical stress are known contributing factors to the development of IBS and FODMAP intolerance as well.

So, what should you do now? If you're struggling with gut problems like IBS, here are some practical ways to start taking action:

1. Try out a low-FODMAP diet.

It has been estimated that around 75% of people struggling with IBS symptoms improve with a low-FODMAP diet. Focus on eating vegetables, fruits, and clean meats that are not on the high-FODMAP list and see if your symptoms improve. The good news is that many people can slowly start reintroducing some of these foods over time as their gut heals.

2. Consider comprehensive GI labs.

Here are a few tests you might want to ask your doctor about:

Lactulose breath test: FODMAP intolerance is linked to small intestinal bacterial overgrowth (also known as SIBO). This lab measures the gases, methane, and hydrogen released by the bacterial overgrowth.

Microbiome stool test: IBS is also associated with an increase in pathogenic (bad) bacteria. By measuring the levels of good and bad bacteria, this will help you understand your unique microbiome issues.

Leaky gut blood lab: If you haven't checked for leaky gut during your gluten-free week, it's time to do this now. In fact, by measuring the antibodies to occludin and zonulin, the proteins that control gut lining permeability, you can assess leaky gut syndrome, which is common with IBS.

3. Consider food allergy labs.

If you're having an intolerance to FODMAPs, it's likely there is an underlying food allergy or intolerance. A true **food allergy** causes an immune system reaction that can affect numerous organs in the body. In contrast, **food intolerance** symptoms are often limited to digestive problems.

4. Manage stress.

Ever wondered why people often have gut problems when they are nervous or stressed? It's because of the gut-brain connection. In fact, **stress alters the gut flora significantly** and research suggests that stress can lead to an overgrowth of certain types of bacteria and decrease the diversity in the microbiome.

5. Take probiotics.

Yes, again. A combination of *Bifidobacteria*, *Enterococcus,* and *Lactobacillus* has been shown as effective in improving irritable bowel syndrome.

TRY: LOW FODMAP WEEK

There are a few gut-healing protocols available today. The one I use is the one I shared in the previous chapter: Remove, Replenish, and Repair. You can also look into the GAPS diet or the specific carbohydrate diet, although they don't really restore your gut health, so I would still recommend a gut-healing protocol while following these diets, so you can treat the cause and not just eliminate the triggers.

1. Remove

Most of the high-FODMAP foods are actually 'healthy foods' for most people, but even when it comes to natural foods, what works for one person may not be right for another. I recommend trying to stick with a low-FODMAP diet for a couple of weeks and see if you feel any better.

Here are the foods that should be avoided, or severely limited, if you have IBS symptoms while you heal your gut.

AVOID THESE FOODS

Vegetable and legumes:

- Garlic
- Onions
- Broccoli
- Asparagus
- Cabbage, common and red
- Beans e.g. black, broad, kidney, lima, soya
- Carrots
- Cauliflower
- Cabbage, savoy
- Celery (less than 5cm stalk)
- Mangetout
- Chickpeas (¼ cup max)
- Corn (½ cob max)
- Mushrooms
- Peas
- Zucchini
- Scallions/spring onions (white part)

Fruit:

Fructose, one of the FODMAP sugars, is one of the more common intolerances and is often found in people with recurring stomach pain and bloating. Try to limit – if not eliminate completely — your fruit consumption. Especially, steer clear of:

- Apples
- Apricots
- Avocados
- Blackberries
- Grapefruits
- Mangoes

- Peaches
- Pears
- Plums
- Raisins
- Sultanas
- Watermelons

Meats:

- Chorizos
- Sausages

- Processed meats

Bread, cereal, grains, and pasta:

- Barley
- Bran
- Couscous

Gnocchi

Granola

Muesli

Nuts:

- Cashews
- Pistachios

Milk:

- Cow's milk
- Goat's milk
- Rice milk
- Sheep's milk
- Soymilk made with soybeans (made with soy protein is okay)

Dairy:

- Buttermilk
- Cream
- Custard
- Greek yogurt
- Ice cream
- Sour cream
- Yogurt
- Cream cheese
- Ricotta cheese

Condiments:

- Hummus dip
- Jam (mixed berries)
- Pasta sauce (cream-based)
- Relish
- Tzatziki dip

Sweeteners:

- Agave
- High fructose corn syrup (HFCS)
- Honey
- Inulin
- Isomalt
- Maltitol
- Mannitol
- Sorbitol
- Xylitol

Drinks:

- Coconut water
- Apple juice
- Pear juice
- Mango juice
- Sodas with HFCS
- Fennel tea

I know you're probably thinking, *Ugh, I pretty much can't eat anything.* Don't panic! To eat without feeling deprived, while still falling within the scope of the low FODMAP diet, stick to this protocol: protein + fat + veggies.

2. Replenish

With FODMAP-intolerance blood tests, you can find out which of the enzymes you need to replenish.

3. Repair

The goal with treating a FODMAP intolerance is not to remove the foods forever, but to heal the gut, so that you can eventually reintroduce these foods to your diet. Providing the nutrients necessary to help the gut repair itself is essential. The protocol to follow to repair your gut is the same one as the previous chapter so carry on with that, following the instructions.

BOTTOM LINE: Millions of people live with undiagnosed bouts of bloating, constipation, and diarrhea, and consider it normal. These symptoms are also known as IBS and can have a serious impact on your quality of life, but it can go beyond bathroom problems. Because of the gut-brain connection, as many as 90% of people with IBS also have psychiatric disorders, including panic disorders, generalized anxiety disorders, and major depression.

If you suffer with IBS and eliminating gluten did not solve your issue, you might want to try a low FODMAP diet for at least a month. FODMAP means foods with fermentable sugars, which are not completely absorbed in the gastrointestinal tract and can easily ferment, causing gas, pain, and diarrhea. A good starting point is to eliminate these foods completely from your diet and see how your body reacts. In the meantime, it's also a good idea to continue to repair your gut with the same protocol I suggested in the previous chapter. Always remember to consult your physician before taking any supplements.

CHECK-IN QUESTIONS

How were your energy levels on a scale of 1 to 10?

Did you feel fatigued or sluggish?

Can you think clearly?

Did you feel tired?

Did you feel bloated?

Did you have headaches? (If yes, how many?)

Did you go to the bathroom regularly?

Is your skin clear?

Did you have cravings?

Did you binge?

Did you eat or snack compulsively or mindlessly?

Is your sleep regular?

Did you have trouble concentrating or brain fog?

Did you suffer with mood swings?

Did you ever feel anxious, fearful, or nervous?

Did you feel physically weak?

Did you get sick?

Did you have bad breath?

Did you have heartburn?

Did you have stomach or intestinal pain?

Did you experience ringing in your ears?

Did you feel the need to urinate urgently or frequently?

Did you have pain or aches in your muscles and joints?

Did you feel stiff or limited in your movements?

"Come here you beautiful cup of coffee and lie to me about how much I am going to get done today."

WEEK 9

IS COFFEE MAKING YOU TIRED?

Have you ever gone a day without your morning cup of Jolt? Although I am a big fan of coffee – duh, I'm Italian, how could I not like espresso? – when it comes down to how it affects people's health, I have realized that this can be a controversial topic. Depending on who you ask, it is either a super healthy beverage or incredibly harmful. The truth is that I used to find this subject to be as confusing as anyone, but after a lot of research, I am able to shine some light on it all.

First up, don't worry - *I'm not going to tell you to stop drinking coffee!* In fact, if you love coffee, keep drinking it because it actually has lots of potential health benefits. What I'm going to show you in this chapter is how to get the benefits without the drawbacks. And it all comes down to how you use it.

So, let's start with the good news: Coffee consumption has been linked to numerous health benefits. Research is considering the protective or preventative properties of coffee for the following conditions, among others:

- Lowering risk of cardiovascular disease

- Lowering risk of diabetes

- Protecting the liver

- Promoting longevity

- Decreasing cancer risk

- Protecting the skin

- Reducing the risk of multiple sclerosis (MS)

- Preventing gout

- Supporting gut health

While all of this sounds great so far, unfortunately assuming that drinking coffee every day is great for you is wrong. Let me explain why very simply.

You see, if you consume coffee every day, *it will cause you to feel tired and sleepy.* By consuming coffee on a daily basis, you will spend most of your life in a *poorer mood, with lower energy and worse mental and physical performance* than if you were not drinking coffee. Even it feels like the caffeine is taking you to new heights, it is not.

What's actually happening is that the habitual caffeine consumption has *lowered your baseline energy level*, causing you to feel sleepy and tired, and you're just giving yourself a boost back up to what used to be your *normal level of function without caffeine*.

So basically, you made yourself dependent on caffeine just to function normally! Pretty crazy, right?

There's a recent study from researchers at Johns Hopkins University on the topic. If you want to know more about this, there is an online article that explains it thoroughly called *Why Does Coffee Make Me Tired?* at theenergyblueprint.com. Or for now, just take my word for it.

Additionally, if you suffer with obesity, anxiety, insomnia, lack of energy, sugar cravings, or you cannot go a day without coffee, here are a few reasons for you to reconsider your coffee habits:

- Evidence from recent studies has linked caffeine use with insulin resistance, adrenal exhaustion, liver and kidney problems, thyroid issues, and a sugar-craving cycle that seems unbreakable. Even a casual consumption of caffeinated beverages has been shown to increase the risk of heart disease.

- Too much caffeine — seven or more cups of coffee a day — can induce dizziness, nausea, headache, muscle tension, sleep disturbances, irregular heartbeat, anxiety attacks, severe drowsiness, ringing in the ears, diarrhea, vomiting, difficulty breathing, and even convulsions.

- Besides caffeine, the chemical laden creamers and sugars (artificial or not) that are usually added, make drinking coffee harmful.

Here's the important part: The only people who are actually getting a ***real lift*** from coffee are those who do not consume it regularly. Only these people will get a boost in their mood, energy, and mental and physical performance. If you drink it all the time, you will not get any benefit. Instead, you will get caffeine fatigue.

However, getting off coffee is not that simple…

ADDICTION

The problem with coffee is that caffeine works on the same parts of the brain as amphetamines, cocaine, and heroin, creating a full-on addiction to it. In fact, caffeine increases dopamine levels in your brain, which is the neurotransmitter that activates the pleasure centers. Your body and brain naturally want to feel good, so when dopamine levels rise, your brain associates the increased happiness feeling with coffee, which will cause you to want more. Besides, once the adrenaline leaves your system, you will feel more fatigued and depressed than before you had the coffee, which will cause you to reach out for another cup. And here you are, looped into this wild addiction.

What's worse is that the cost of a caffeine addiction can add up to thousands of dollars a year that could be saved if you quit. Below I have listed the average cost of just one beverage per day for a number of coffee shop or store-bought products. Multiply the numbers by the number of cups you have each day and it adds up quickly.

- Grande Starbucks Latte: $3.65 a day | $26 a week | **$1,332 a year**

- Monster Energy Drink: $3 a day | $21 a week | **$1,095 a year**

- Home-brewed coffee: $0.71 a day | $5 per week | **$259 a year**

- K-cups: $0.65 a day | $4.55 a week | **$237 a year**

- 5-Hour Energy: $3 a day | $21 a week | **$1,095 a year**

Besides getting you addicted by increasing dopamine levels, caffeine stimulates the pituitary gland, which releases a hormone that tells your adrenals to produce the stress hormones adrenaline and cortisol. In other words, you are triggering exactly the same kind of stress response that your body uses when you are in imminent physical danger.

Adrenaline is responsible for the heart beating faster and the blood vessels diverting blood from surface areas to our muscles. Consequently, your blood pressure rises, and stomach function slows, as does your body's ability to absorb vitamins, minerals, and other valuable materials vital for your health. So, if you are working hard to get all the necessary vitamins and minerals into your diet, drinking coffee is sabotaging all your efforts.

Cortisol, a stress hormone naturally present in the body, when chronically elevated, can have deleterious effects on weight, immune function — limiting the ability of your immune system to fight infection — and makes chronic disease risk higher.

As you can see, there is anything but balance in this caffeinated cycle. We're slaves to it. And this detox is all about restoring balance within our body.

HOW TO GET THE BENEFITS FROM COFFEE

The bad news is that you have to give your brain a complete break from caffeine for several weeks. I recommend at least five to six weeks without coffee. The good news is that once you cleanse your system, you can consume coffee again in moderation, as long as it's on and off. For example, drink coffee for one or two days, then take a break for two to three days. Or use it for two weeks and then go off for two weeks.

I know, I know. Giving up your morning cup of coffee or caffeinated soda might sound like a joke. I've been there myself and it's tough, but this little task is an important part of detoxing your body and will help your energy levels.

This coffee-free phase does not have to carry on forever, but do give this a try, especially if you suffer from insomnia, anxiety, a lack of energy, indigestion, acid reflux, or Type II diabetes. Especially with insomnia, the NSF has estimated that anything beyond a cup of coffee or two sodas a day may start to affect sleep. Cutting caffeine is a great way to get your sleep schedule back on track.

TRY: EASE OFF COFFEE WEEK

I know it may be daunting but please don't discount it before you read it.

YOU CAN'T GO COLD TURKEY

Quitting coffee should be done with care, as your body will react immediately and forcefully to its absence. You could experience short-term withdrawal symptoms from caffeine, but they are generally gone within a week. I know this could make the idea of kicking coffee out of your diet for good too hard to contemplate, but please be gentle with yourself and try to see it through.

That said, I have created a protocol to follow to avoid withdrawal symptoms, based on my personal experience. I've refined it through the years after applying this method with my clients.

DAYS 1 to 4: Go half-caf first

Drink your usual number of cups of coffee, subbing half of your regular coffee dosage with decaf. In addition, drink a cup of regular water, hot or cold, for every cup of coffee you drink. Continue with these half-mixes daily for the first four days.

DAYS 5 to 8: Alternate half-caf and decaf

It's time to make the switch to a full cup of decaf coffee. The ratio is one fully decaf coffee for every half-caf coffee. For example, if you drink two cups a day, make one cup half caf + half decaf, and the other cup all decaf. If you drink four cups a day, make two cups half caf + half decaf, and two cups full decaf. And so forth.

In addition, drink a cup of regular water, hot or cold, for every cup of coffee you drink. You can also try tea to help with energy. If you need something warm and soothing, try green tea, yerba mate, ginseng, ginger, licorice, or ginkgo biloba.

Continue with these half-mixes daily for the following four days.

DAY 9: Decaf time!

Congratulations, you are doing great! It has been over a week since you started reducing caffeine from your life. You should already be starting to feel better.

If you are used to consuming only two cups a day, it's time to cut down to drink only decaffeinated coffee.

'Swiss water process' decaffeinated coffee is the best, as it is processed with a non-chemical method of removing caffeine from the beans.

NOTE: If you consume more than four cups a day, continue every four days to switch one cup of caffeinated coffee to a full decaf until you are drinking only decaf. In addition, drink a cup of regular water, hot or cold, for every cup of coffee you drink.

DAY 12: Goodbye coffee

It's time to lower the actual amount of cups of coffee you drink. The goal is to have no coffee at all. Try to substitute coffee with tea. The best teas for energy are green tea, yerba mate, ginseng, ginger, licorice, and ginkgo biloba.

TIPS FOR TRANSITIONING

I invite you to get creative for the next four coffee-free weeks. Experiment with different teas, add milk substitutes (almond, cashew, coconut, or rice milk) and a little raw honey to really make it enjoyable.

Some of my favorite combos are:

- Green tea (alone or with almond milk and organic raw unfiltered honey)

- Chai tea with rice milk (optional organic raw unfiltered honey)

- Peppermint with almond milk (optional organic raw unfiltered honey)

- Yerba mate with almond or rice milk and a little organic raw unfiltered honey

- Black tea with almond milk and organic raw unfiltered honey

- Breakfast tea with almond or rice milk

- Matcha latte with almond milk

Just keep in mind that rice milk is usually sweetened, so you don't need to add in honey or any other sweetener. That would be too much sugar and you know what that means!

Creating your own ritual with tea is a great way to carve out some quiet time during the day and take a break for a self-nurturing practice. Gather items that are appealing as well as calming to you. Some ideas could be a teapot, two or three teacups or mugs, teaspoons, and a small collection of different herbal teas for different moods. Choose a special place for all your tea items. Then find 15 to 30 minutes during the day to sit down with your tea. Enjoy it with a friend and some conversation, a journal for reflection, or a good book. Try to put on some calming music and sit quietly while you sip your tea. Personally, I love to listen to Buddha Bar or Nirinjan Kaur's station on Pandora while sitting on something comfortable (possibly furry or fluffy), reading something or just starring outside, letting my thoughts run wild.

Perhaps creating a ritual of a tea break mid-morning and/or mid-afternoon can help revive the usual three o'clock energy lag at the office.

Other ways to energize your body are:

- Drink water and a cap of apple cider vinegar

- Walk (for 10 minutes)

- Do 30 jumping jacks

- Stretch your muscles (for example, with yoga)

- Supplement with these herbs or roots in natural form or as tea:

Gotu kola: Decreases fatigue and/or depression and stimulates central nervous system.

Lavender: Relieves stress and headaches.

Maca: Increases energy and supports the immune system.

Ginseng: For energy and resilience. Ginseng is prescribed by herbalists to boost your resilience to stress and stress-related fatigue. Other beneficial effects are boosting the immune system, helping jetlag, and potentially increasing fertility.

Ginger: To uplift the spirit. Ginger stimulates the circulatory system, helping to clear the mind and stimulate the brain. It is very beneficial for the stomach and is an effective natural remedy for all forms of nausea — from morning sickness to travel sickness.

Licorice: Licorice root has been described as 'the universal herb'. It has many benefits, but most importantly, supports adrenal gland function and mitigates endocrine exhaustion. For anyone suffering from low energy levels, licorice works to restore adrenal glands that have been worn out by too much stress. It is also an anti-stress mood booster and stabilizes blood-sugar levels. By drinking licorice tea, you won't experience the 'energy crash' that has you reaching for coffee and a donut in the late afternoon.

Ginkgo biloba: Very popular in Chinese medicine for its ability to increase blood-flow to the brain, ginkgo biloba improves concentration and memory retention naturally. It enhances energy levels generally and stimulates your circulatory system, which helps with varicose veins, cold hands and feet, and fatigue. It can raise blood pressure if taken in large quantities over time, so avoid if you have high blood pressure.

Rosehip: This traditional tea is a wonderful source of vitamin C, giving it anti-aging effects and young-looking skin support. It has a refreshing, berry-like taste and is a great way to start your morning.

REINTRODUCING COFFEE...

Coffee needs to become something you are gifting yourself and not just a daily habit. I like to treat myself to a cappuccino every now and then as a reward for my hard work or when I can't seem to wake up in the morning. Just like everything else, when sourcing your coffee, only drink high quality coffee and make sure it is:

Organic: Coffee is one of the most heavily sprayed crops for pesticides. Imported beans can be coated with unregulated pesticides used in foreign countries. Any coffee you consume should be organic, pesticide-free coffee.

Whole bean: You'll want to purchase coffee in whole-bean form and then grind it yourself to prevent rancidity. Pre-ground coffee may be rancid by the time you drink it.

Dark roast: It's often the case that foods with the darkest pigments also offer the most robust benefits to health. Dark roast coffee, such as French roast, the kind used to make espresso, or Turkish coffee, is no exception. Research in *Molecular Nutrition & Food Research* found that dark roast coffee restored blood levels of the antioxidants vitamin E and glutathione more effectively than light roast coffee.

Black: Drink your coffee or cappuccino black without sugar or cream. If you add sugar, you'll certainly ruin any of the benefits discussed above by spiking your insulin levels. And if you opt for a dairy-free cappuccino, make sure that the milk substitute of your choice is unsweetened especially when ordering it out!

Further, if you use a drip coffee maker, be sure to use non-bleached filters. The bright white ones, which most people use, are chlorine bleached and some of this chlorine will be extracted from the filter during the brewing process. They are also full of dangerous disinfection byproducts like dioxin.

BOTTOM LINE: Although coffee has some health benefits, like with everything else, too much of a good thing can be bad. One cup of coffee a day is not going to kill you, but it can make you more tired than normal. Coffee should be consumed as a treat or to serve its purpose rather than a daily habit but breaking free from a caffeine addiction can be really challenging. By following my protocol, you should be able to gently detach yourself from the disruptive cycle of caffeine. A great way to transition out of coffee is to substitute it with tea. There are many different teas you can try that will help you relax, and gain energy and mental clarity. Follow my protocol to get yourself off this addiction and try to stick to a caffeine-free lifestyle at least a month.

When you reintroduce coffee, it is as a treat or as a tool. And remember don't drink it every day, but every couple of days. Make sure to source the highest quality coffee, following the guidelines.

CHECK-IN QUESTIONS

How were your energy levels on a scale of 1 to 10?

Did you feel fatigued or sluggish?

Can you think clearly?

Did you feel tired?

Did you feel bloated?

Did you have headaches? (If yes, how many?)

Did you go to the bathroom regularly?

Is your skin clear?

Did you have cravings?

Did you binge?

Did you eat or snack compulsively or mindlessly?

Is your sleep regular?

Did you have trouble concentrating? (Foggy brain)

Did you suffer with mood swings?

Did you ever feel anxious, fearful, or nervous?

Did you feel physically weak?

Did you get sick?

Did you have bad breath?

Did you have heartburn?

Did you have stomach or intestinal pain?

Did you experience ringing in your ears?

Did you feel the need to urinate urgently or frequently?

Did you have pain or aches in your muscles and joints?

Did you feel stiff or limited in your movements?

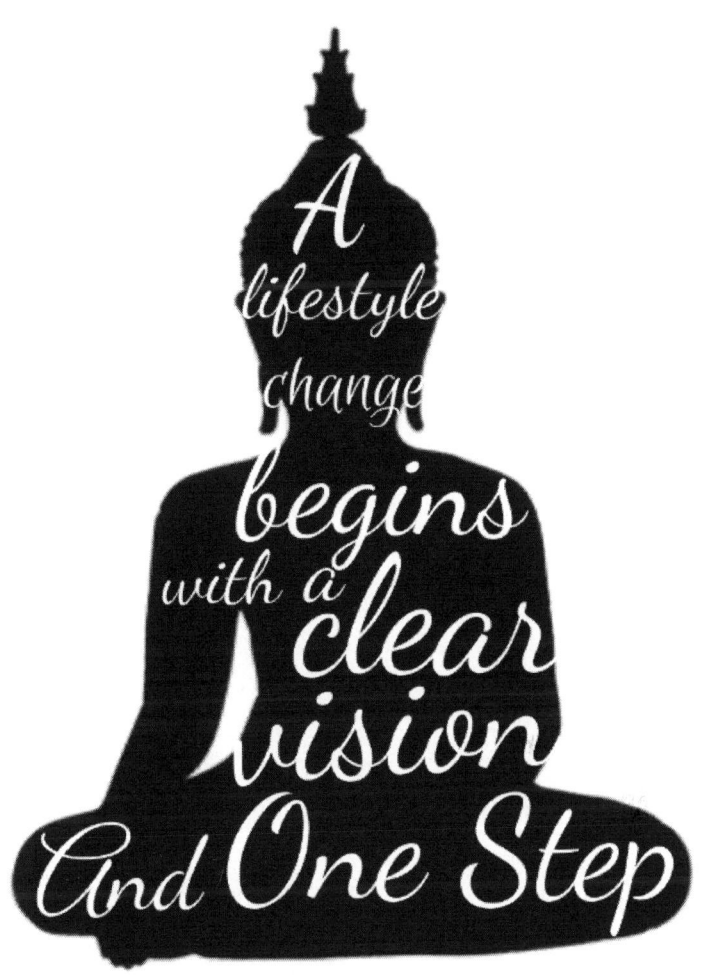

A lifestyle change begins with a clear vision And One Step

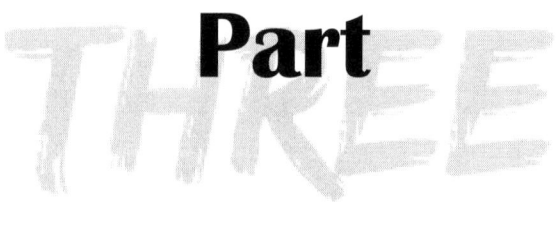

Part THREE

ADDRESSING LIFESTYLE

We're reaching the last stretch of our journey together. I hope you've taken plenty of value from this book.

So far, we have covered your mindset, then addressed your body through nutrition. Now it's time to touch on the topic of recharging your soul. Your mind-body-soul connection is what makes you truly healthy, so this book would be incomplete if we didn't mention it.

Let's take a look.

*"Please Note:
hitting the gym to
release stress
is not nearly as
effective as hitting the
people that caused
the stress to begin with."*

WEEK 10

IS YOUR LIFESTYLE MAKING YOU FAT?

Stress is our physical, emotional, and behavioral *reaction* to any demand or change that we believe challenges our capacity to cope. It's a part of life, which means we will experience stressful moments no matter what. But that's not necessarily a bad thing.

BENEFITS OF STRESS

While stress affects everyone in different ways, it's important to recognize that stress can be beneficial. In fact, we *need some stress* in our lives.

Stress is a vital warning system, the body's natural response to unexpected or dangerous situations that advises you on what to do. When faced with something unusual (a challenge or stressor), your body activates resources to protect you either by preparing you to stay and fight or to get away as fast as possible (the well-known fight-or-flight response).

This response creates a large quantity of the chemicals cortisol, adrenaline, and noradrenaline, which cause an increase in our heart rate and blood pressure, heightened muscle preparedness, and sharper vision, hearing, sweating, and alertness.

In small doses, this has many advantages:

- Helps you accomplish tasks more efficiently
- Boosts your memory
- Helps you meet daily challenges
- Motivates you to reach your goals

The body's stress-response system is usually self-limiting. Once a perceived threat has passed, hormone levels return to normal. As adrenaline and cortisol levels drop, your heart rate and blood pressure return to baseline levels, and other systems resume their regular activities.

So, it all seems good, right? Wrong.

When stressors are always present and you feel constantly under attack, that fight-or-flight reaction stays turned on. If you don't learn to control stress, your body's natural stress response will have a significant impact on your immune system, brain chemistry, blood-sugar levels, hormonal balance, and much more.

In fact, the downsides of the fight-or-flight response is the release of cortisol, the primary stress hormone, which increases sugars (glucose) in the bloodstream, enhances your brain's use of glucose and increases the availability of substances that repair tissues.

Cortisol also curbs functions that would be non-essential or detrimental in a fight-or-flight situation. It alters immune system responses and suppresses the digestive system, the reproductive system, and growth processes. This complex natural alarm system also communicates with the regions of your brain that control mood, motivation, and fear.

Although stress is key for survival, too much stress can be detrimental. Emotional stress that stays around for weeks or months can weaken the immune system and cause high blood pressure, autoimmune illnesses, digestive issues, fatigue, depression, anxiety, weight gain, and even heart disease. In particular, too much epinephrine can be harmful to your heart as it can change the arteries and how the cells are able to regenerate.

So, it's important to manage stress, prevent negative stress levels, and speak up if you are feeling overwhelmed.

RECOGNIZING YOUR STRESS SYMPTOMS

Symptoms of too much stress can be physical, emotional, mental, and behavioral. I know it may be tough to tell if you're experiencing good or bad stress, but your body will alert you when your system is overwhelmed with the following warning signs:

- Inability to concentrate or complete tasks

- Get sick more often

- Body aches

- Other illnesses like autoimmune diseases flare up

- Headaches

- Irritability

- Trouble falling sleeping or staying awake

- Changes in appetite

- Trouble concentrating

- Racing thoughts

- Memory problems

- Sadness

- Changes in sleep or appetite

- Angrier or more anxious than usual

SLEEP AND STRESS

Getting a good night of sleep is an important part of detoxing — and overall wellbeing — just as nutrition and exercise are. Sleep affects our focus, mood, productivity, mental, and physical health. Yet many of us go through life completely sleep-deprived. According to a 2013 International Bedroom Poll, half the population in the United States sleeps less than the seven recommended hours per night during the week, which is the minimum amount of hours your body needs to restore itself. Chances are you fall into this sleep-deprived category.

During sleep hours, your brain resets and gets sharper. It consolidates your memories and what you learned while awake. Meanwhile, your body clears out toxins, lowers your stress by dropping cortisol levels, releases hormones that directly impact your growth and metabolism, and your immune system gets stronger.

The consequences of not getting enough sleep are extremely serious. Besides a lack of focus, low energy, and moodiness, sleep deprivation leads to a higher risk of heart attack, strokes, Type II diabetes, cancer, and obesity, as well as depression, irritability, and anxiety.

You may be thinking that I'm exaggerating here; that you can function just fine after four to six hours of sleep. I am sure you know someone who feels exactly the same too. What you – or they — don't realize is that it's likely that you are being kept alert by adrenaline, which consequently stimulates norepinephrine and cortisol, all stress hormones, rather than being awake because you are truly rested and energized. This is what causes you to sabotage all your weight loss efforts along with seriously compromising your health.

Put simply, and to inspire you to make the changes necessary to ensure you get the most blissful seven hours of sleep (minimum) per night, here's how this works:

Adrenaline is a naturally occurring hormone released during a time of stress, anger, or fear. This hormone is meant to help us survive a potential emergency, and it's a crucial part of the body's fight-or-flight response. Produced by the adrenal gland after receiving a message from the brain that a stressful situation has presented itself, this hormone is responsible for the immediate reactions we have when facing danger or under stress.

At the same time, your brain also releases norepinephrine, another hormone that makes you become more aware, awake, and focused. This hormone also helps to shift blood flow away from areas where it might not be so crucial, like the skin, toward more essential areas, like the muscles, so you can flee the stressful scene. Finally, cortisol gets activated.

Cortisol helps to maintain fluid balance in our body and blood pressure in a dangerous (stressful) situation, while regulating some body functions that aren't crucial in the moment. The bodily functions that usually get shut down are the reproductive drive, immunity, digestion, and growth. In survival mode, these changes can be lifesaving. But when the body continuously releases cortisol, it will then suppress the immune system, increase blood pressure, and blood sugar, decrease libido, produce acne, contribute to obesity, and more.

This is why if you are not hitting the minimum of seven hours of sleep per night –which is the minimum your body needs to regenerate — you are not only putting your health at risk but also sabotaging all your efforts to stay healthy and potentially lose weight.

ARE YOU SLEEP-DEPRIVED?

So, how do you know whether you are functioning from pure energy or using the energy that comes from your stress hormones? Here's a little assessment to help you decode your body's signals and determine if it's asking for more sleep.

How quickly do you fall asleep when your head hits the pillow?

It should take you between 10 and 20 minutes to drift off into your first stage of sleep. If you fall asleep within 5 to 10 minutes, your body is telling you that you are experiencing moderate sleep deprivation. If it takes you less than five minutes to fall asleep, your body is trying to tell you that you're extremely sleep-deprived.

Do you need to nap during the day?

Although napping is a cultural norm in many countries, if you find yourself nodding off because you are too tired during the day, you can consider yourself sleep-deprived. Your brain simply can't function without more sleep and you need to rest.

Are you often forgetful?

As mentioned above, it is during sleep hours that your brain consolidates memories. A lack of deep sleep, therefore, could be negatively affecting your ability to create and store memories, both long- and short-term.

Are you having a hard time losing weight?

According to a 2004 study, people who sleep less than six hours a day were almost 30% more likely to become obese than those who slept seven to nine hours. Sleep deprivation also often stimulates an increase in appetite and makes you crave foods high in fat and carbs. Additionally, sleep deprivation has been associated with lower levels of growth hormone, which may translate into a slower metabolism. So, if you are trying to lose weight, not sleeping enough could be sabotaging your weight loss efforts.

How is your sex drive?

A side effect of lack and/or poor sleeping habits is also that testosterone levels can drop, which can cause a reduction in libido in both men and women. Of course, feeling sleepy, tired, having low energy, and being cranky also causes you to have a lower sex drive, but if you find yourself with no drive for an extended period of time and can't quite pinpoint why, you'll definitely want to improve your sleep routine.

TIPS FOR GOOD SLEEP

Hopefully by now, you are convinced that your body — especially your brain — needs sleep. Now, to ensure you get the most peaceful, restful, and deep hours of sleep each and every night, here are my top 10 suggestions:

Try to get between seven and eight hours of sleep each night. This is the good-sleep sweet spot for optimal energy, health, and longevity.

Don't eat foods or drink beverages with caffeine before bedtime. Indeed, try to cut out caffeine after 2pm. Did you know that caffeine — even just one cup or one can of soda — can stay in your system for up to eight hours? In an estimation, the National Sleep Foundation (NSF) discovered that anything beyond 250 milligrams of caffeine in one day may start to affect sleep. As we saw in the chapter about coffee, cutting caffeine in general is a great way to not only get your sleep schedules back on track, but also to have more sustained energy levels throughout the day.

Don't eat for at least one to two hours before going to sleep. Also, focusing on a simple, light meal at the end of the day can ease digestion. Foods such as bananas, dates, figs, nut butters, or yogurt can be calming since they all contain tryptophan, which promotes sleep. At dinner, eat foods containing nutrients that promote sleep, including tryptophan, melatonin, and magnesium, and try to eat a combination of high-quality proteins and complex carbohydrates.

Exercise regularly. People who get daily aerobic activity sleep better and more deeply than sedentary people. It's important, though, not to exercise within an hour or two of bedtime, as this will have the opposite effect.

Go to bed at the same time every night and wake up at the same time every day. We humans are creatures of habit and so are our bodies. A consistent sleep schedule is key, as your body thrives on routine. In fact, with a regular daily schedule – for meals, breaks, sleep, and working out — your various body systems are able to prepare for and anticipate events. For example, your body will become more alert closer to your wake-up time, your digestive systems become activated before your usual mealtime to help you digest food more efficiently, and you start to relax and become sleepier before bedtime. You get the picture.

Having a daily schedule in place will help anchor your underlying daily rhythms so that the body doesn't have to think about them and can focus its attention on healing itself. Going to bed at a different time every night, waking up at different times every morning or hitting the snooze button 80 times will throw your body off its rhythm.

Lower the lights an hour before going to sleep: This will help your brain prepare and accept the upcoming end of day, so it will calm down your thinking. Also, the bulbs in your house emit blue-spectrum light (like sunlight), which suppresses the production of melatonin, a crucial hormone for sleep.

Do not text, email, watch videos, or check social media once you get into bed. The blue light from any electronic device is what keeps your brain active and engaged, making it harder to fall asleep and stay deeply asleep.

Use earplugs to block out street noise or your partner's snoring. I don't think I need to explain this.

If you want to drink alcohol, limit yourself to a glass or two and stop an hour before bed. Believe it or not, even though alcohol might make you pass out fast, it seriously hurts the quality of your sleep. It takes about an hour to break down one glass of alcoholic beverage in your stomach so give yourself the proper time to fully process it before going to bed.

If you like to have something before bed and your glass of wine is too hard to let go, try a cup of chamomile (if you are not allergic to ragweed) or catnip tea. The warm sensation is soothing and helps your body relax. Both these teas have mildly sedating properties, which will help you fall asleep, but there are more sleep aid tea alternatives out there, so do some research.

Do not sleep in on weekends: I know this can sound crazy but sleeping in confuses your body's rhythms, just as much as jetlag does. Sleeping in on the weekend will also make it harder to fall back into your sleeping routine at the start of the week.

Once you wake up in the morning, expose yourself immediately to natural light or sunlight if possible. This signals your body that the day has begun. By doing so, it will cut off the hormones that make you groggy and stimulate the ones that perk you up.

Try to sleep on your left side, as a general guideline. There are many health benefits related to this. Especially when it comes to detox, the left side of your body is the dominant lymphatic side, which is the system that remove toxins and waste from your body. So, by sleeping on your left side you may find out that your body becomes more efficient at removing waste as well as relieving acid reflux.

To help fall asleep, read something in bed, download a guided meditation to relax, or do a few simple restorative yoga poses or stretching techniques before bedtime. (You can find loads on YouTube).

QUIET THE MIND

All of these tricks can help calm your body, quiet your mind, and reset your nervous system. Whatever you choose, try to dedicate at least 20 minutes (an hour would be best) to complete wind-down time.

The two key steps to falling asleep are: relaxing your body and shutting down your busy, uncontrollable mind, or 'the monkey mind' as it's called in Buddhism. This means learning to detach from the uncontrollable thoughts of the day.

Our thoughts, like what we've left undone or forgotten to do, can trigger the release of stress hormones such as cortisol, which elevates many body functions like heart rate, blood pressure, breathing, and body temperature. Cortisol is the same hormone responsible for signaling to your brain that it needs to wake up in the morning. Needless to say, this is the last thing you want to signal your brain before going to bed, right?

Of course, calming your thoughts is easier said than done, especially with our crazy busy lives in this hectic society. After coaching many of my clients, I have come up with a few tricks that should help you unwind before bed and calm this monkey mind of yours. These are a few techniques that can help you when nothing else seems to work.

1. Make a list before bedtime. If you are used to not being able to sleep because you can't stop thinking, or if you wake up in the middle of the night and cannot fall back to sleep because of your thoughts running wild, this exercise is great for you. Before going to bed make two lists: one for your unfinished business from the day and one your to-do list for the next day. By writing down everything you can possibly think of on both lists, your brain should be more at ease to let go of the thoughts and accept that it's time to relax. Then breathe deeply. Fill up your lungs until there is no more space and gently release the breath back out, while repeating in your head 10 times, "I am done for today. I will start again tomorrow."

2. Take a warm bath before bed. This can help particularly if you've had a very stressful day, running around like a hamster on a wheel. In fact, taking a warm bath eases your muscles and your mind. Into the hot tub, pour half a cup of Epsom salts with a few drops of lavender essential oil to maximize the benefits. The magnesium found in Epsom salts is absorbed through the skin and promotes muscle relaxation and cleanses the energy from the day. Soak for 20 minutes.

3. Take relaxation breaks during the day. Try to take at least two 15-minute breaks, one in the morning and one in the afternoon, to relax and sit with your thoughts. *No phones allowed* during this time. This will not only help you keep your body in balance so that you're not in a state of overwhelm by the end of the day, but it will also promote a more relaxed way of thinking.

4. Practice left-nostril breathing. Did you know that left-nostril breathing has a soothing and relaxing effect on the body and mind? In Kundalini yoga, it's a common practice to *take 26 long, slow deep left-nostril breaths* to produce a relaxing effect on the mind and body. How to do it? Very simple. Block off your right nostril with your right thumb and take long slow deep breaths through your left nostril only.

5. Practice the 4-7-8 breathing technique. This breathing exercise is a natural tranquilizer for the nervous system. Unlike tranquilizing drugs that take effect almost immediately, this exercise gains power with repetition and practice. To begin, practice **at least twice a day**, once in the morning and once in the evening. I recommend a minimum of four cycles of breath to a maximum of eight breaths total. You can choose whatever suits you best. It is really simple, takes almost no time, and can be done anywhere. Here's how:

- Place the tip of your tongue against the ridge of tissue behind your upper front teeth. You will keep it there through the entire exercise, including when exhaling.

- Exhale completely through your mouth, making a *whoosh* sound.

- Close your mouth and inhale quietly through your nose to a mental count of **four**.

- Hold your breath for a count of **seven**.

- Exhale audibly and completely through your mouth, making a *whoosh* sound to a count of **eight**.

This is one breath. Now inhale again and repeat the cycle three more times for a total of four breaths.

You can use this technique whenever anything upsetting happens – before you react, or whenever you are aware of internal tension. Use it to help you fall asleep, deal with food cravings, when experiencing moderate anxiety, or any time you feel tense. All my clients who have tried this have had amazing benefits from it. So, if you love it just as much as I do, share it with all your loved ones.

6. Put one or two drops of lavender essential oil on your pillow before going to bed. This will help you relax and reach a deeper state of rest.

7. Try natural remedies. One hour before bed you can try taking one of these:

- 300 to 600 milligrams of passionflower (Passiflora)

- 320 to 480 milligrams of valerian root extract (Valeriana)

- 365 milligrams of magnolia

- 1 to 3 milligrams of melatonin

- 150 to 300 milligrams of magnesium

8. If you wake up in the middle of the night, leave the bedroom and spend 'unpleasant' awake time in another room. Only use the bedroom for sleep, sex, changing clothes, and other pleasant activities, leaving anything stressful outside. This is especially important for people who suffer with insomnia, because by 'hanging out' in the bedroom while distressed, you subconsciously create a relationship with this room as a place of tension and unpleasant moments. If you wake up in the middle of the night and want to work on the computer, read emails, talk on the phone, or watch TV, get out of the bedroom and spend any waking moments elsewhere. By doing so, you will help your brain associate the bedroom with a place of rest, where it can go to disconnect. This will help you relax when entering the room in future.

9. Shift your perspective about sleep. Lots of the time, when someone has not been sleeping well for a while, the fear of not being able to fall asleep is actually what keeps them from falling asleep or not sleeping properly through the night. Other times, the thought of needing a set amount of hours (like the seven or eight recommended) will have the same effect.

If you suffer from insomnia it's likely that when you walk into your bedroom, you feel anxious and uncomfortable at the thought of spending the night tossing and turning. It's time to break this cycle. Like mentioned above, help your brain associate new healthy feelings with your sleep by making a small investment in changing a few things around, so it becomes one of the most inviting rooms in the house, if not the most.

Here are some tips to help you set up your bedroom in a way that is inviting, visually pleasing and comfortable, kind of like those bedrooms in the magazines. A little investment can go a long way.

UPGRADE YOUR BEDROOM

Creating a peaceful environment in which to sleep will entice you to prioritize a good night's sleep.

Make it a distraction-free zone: Declutter your room from everything that does not belong in it — documents, files, boxes, etc. You should only have a bed and bedroom furniture in your bedroom, possibly some clothes. Anything that does not belong in these three categories should be left out. Remove the television, computer, and any other stress-inducing and distracting appliances from your bedroom.

Colors: When you walk into your bedroom, you want to feel really relaxed and restful, almost a little Zen. When choosing bedroom colors to promote sleep — whether for walls, bedding, or accents — think of light blues, earth tones, creamy shades or soft, muted colors instead of bold or bright ones.

Blackouts: Lights shut down your body's production of melatonin, so it is important to sleep with a mask or install blackouts in your bedroom. Blackouts will block up to 99% of light and the honeycomb design absorbs sounds too, ensuring a restful night of sleep.

Clock/alarm: Clocks with blue-toned digits block melatonin production and keep you up. Instead, pick a clock that emits an amber light or one of the old-fashioned analog ones.

Temperature: Setting your thermostat between 65 and 71 degrees helps you reach that perfect core temperature that allows you to sleep more easily and deeply.

Pets out: I am a huge supporter of pets. (I have a Pomeranian and he is the love of my life!) But it has been proven that almost a quarter of the people who suffer with insomnia sleep with their pet. You see, as much as our hairy friends are like our babies and we can't live without them, the hair, the tossing, the turning, the occasional snoring, and our inability to properly move in our beds is what keeps people from getting a good night's sleep. So, if you suffer with poor sleep, leave your pet out. I know the transition won't be fun for either of you, but it will be worth it in the long run. You can help 'sweeten' the deal by putting a treat on their bed outside your bedroom.

Upgrade the mattress: Mattresses accumulate sweat, oil, and dust mites so you do want to replace yours after five to ten years. Look for one made with natural rubber so it will discourage the mites and absorb motions. If you can, try to not go cheap. Personally, I love the Casper or Tempur-pedic brands.

Pillow: The way you lie down every night can determine which pillow is best for you. The right pillow will keep your head in a neutral position, which will vary depending on your sleeping position and whether you suffer from allergies:

- **ALLERGIES:** Choose synthetic materials instead of down and feathers.

- **IF YOU SLEEP ON YOUR BACK:** Look for a pillow with a firm latex edge to support and relax your neck and a soft downy area in the middle that lets you rest your head in a neutral position.

- **IF YOU SLEEP ON YOUR STOMACH:** Choose a thinner flatter cushion.

- **IF YOU SLEEP ON YOUR SIDE:** A plumper pillow fills up the space between the neck and shoulder keeping your spine aligned. Try a small pillow in between your knees as well, so your hips will not get inflamed.

TRY: MANAGE YOUR STRESS WEEK

Stress and its triggers are different for everyone. Certain people, places, or situations might produce high levels of stress for you. So, the first thing you need to learn is to identify your triggers.

IDENTIFY YOUR TRIGGERS

Think about what causes you stress, and brainstorm solutions. If, for example, there are friends or social situations that cause extreme stress, you may want to avoid them when you are already feeling tense or overwhelmed. If any type of performance stresses you out (for example, public speaking, a presentation, etc.), you want to **practice a lot**, until you feel comfortable. If it's a deadline that makes you tense, you may want to make sure you organize yourself properly. If you struggle with time management, try not to over-commit yourself. Jot down everything you need to do in a calendar or a task management app or program. Prioritize your list and break projects into single steps or actions. And remember to focus on one task at a time, as multitasking rarely works.

You get the idea. Find solutions to your stressors.

FOODS TO FIGHT STRESS

Here's some good news to keep in mind the next time you're stressed out: Eating may help you stay calm. But here's the thing: I'm not talking about stuffing yourself with your typical go-to comfort food. Mac and cheese, pizza, or fries will only leave you feeling guilty and even more anxious. Instead, feed your face with one (or more) of these foods to feel at ease fast.

- **Asparagus:** High in folate, which is essential for keeping your cool. I like it steamed, then added to salads. I also love it broiled until crisp.

- **Avocados:** These creamy fruits stress-proof your body. Rich in glutathione, a substance that specifically blocks intestinal absorption of certain fats that cause oxidative damage, avocados also contain lutein, beta-carotene, vitamin E, and more folate than any other fruit.

- **Berries:** All berries, including strawberries, raspberries, and blackberries, are rich in vitamin C, which has been shown to be helpful in combating stress.

- **Cashews:** abundant in vitamin B6 — which helps produce serotonin, the feel-good hormone — they are also a good source of magnesium, which plays a significant role in stabilizing energy as well as regulating the nervous system.

- **Red peppers:** While oranges get all the vitamin C hype, red peppers have about twice as much (95 vs. 50 mg per half-cup serving). In a study in *Psychopharmacology*, people who took high doses of vitamin C before engaging in stress-inducing activities (an oral presentation followed by solving math problems aloud) had lower blood pressure and recovered faster from the cortisol surge than those who got a placebo.

- **Omegas:** To keep your wits about you when life gets hairy, you need omega-3s, especially DHA. You won't get the same mood boost from the omega-3s (ALA) in flax, walnuts, or soy, though, so shoot for about two servings a week of wild salmon or other oily fish and/or grass-fed, organic beef, or talk to your doctor about a daily omega supplement.

- **Dark chocolate (75% or higher):** There's evidence that, in moderation, chocolate does actually make you feel better. Dark chocolate, in particular, is known to lower blood pressure, adding to a feeling of calm.

- **Eat plenty of spinach, seeds, beans, and brown rice:** These are all rich in stress-busting magnesium, which helps regulate cortisol and blood pressure. And since magnesium gets flushed out of the body when you're stressed, it's crucial to get enough.

- **Sip on tea:** Doesn't the thought of sipping a mug of hot tea sound calming already? A study from University College London discovered that tea drinkers de-stressed faster and had lower cortisol levels! So, schedule in some teatime: chamomile, green tea, and black tea all work, so pick your favorite.

- **Garlic:** Because stress weakens the immune system, we need friends like garlic, which can toughen it back up.

- **Oatmeal:** Talk about comfort food! A complex carbohydrate, oatmeal causes your brain to produce serotonin, a feel-good chemical. Not only does serotonin have antioxidant properties, it also creates a soothing feeling that helps overcome stress.

- **Get a good probiotic, possibly one with *Lactobacillus rhamnosus*:** One of the most renowned health doctors, Dr. Mercola says, "This probiotic was found to have a marked effect on GABA levels in certain brain regions and lowered the stress-induced hormone corticosterone, resulting in reduced anxiety- and depression-related behavior."

- **QUICK NOTE ON CRAVINGS:** When stressed out, your cravings will increase as a side effect of cortisol. Although you will naturally crave processed carbohydrates and sugar (especially women), try to avoid them, along with gluten and processed foods in general. There is plenty of scientific evidence that you can find on this topic, if you are interested in reading further.

OTHER STRESS RELIEF

Relaxation techniques are a huge help in calming you down, boosting your mood, and fighting illness. Try a variety of techniques to see what works for you and schedule a relaxation break every day.

- Massage

- Meditation

- Bubble bath

- Slow beat music, relaxing sounds

- Hobbies/distractions

- Progressive muscle relaxation therapy

- Visualization

- Journaling/reading

Certain herbs can help fight the symptoms of stress too. See the Natural Remedies section at the back of the book for more.

BREATHING: Inhaling and exhaling slowly can help ease symptoms such as rapid heartbeat. The extra oxygen can help clear your mind and gives you time to sort out your thoughts. Try meditative breathing:

Sit straight up in a chair with your feet comfortably on the floor and your hands in your lap, resting on your thighs. Close your eyes and just be aware of your breath. Are you breathing mostly from your chest, in short, shallow breaths? Begin to deepen your breath by slowly inflating your belly and chest for a count of four. Hold each breath for seven counts and exhale for a count of eight. Slowly begin again. Do this 10 times.

NATURAL MEDICINE: Adaptogens are a unique class of healing plants that help balance, restore, and protect the body. According to naturopath, Edward Wallace, an adaptogen doesn't have a specific action; it helps you respond to any influence or stressor, normalizing your physiological functions. The best ones are ginseng, holy basil, ashwagandha, astragalus root, licorice root, rhodiola, cordycep reishi, shiitake and maitake mushrooms.

IMPORTANT NOTE: As always, you should discuss any new supplements or medications with your doctor before beginning a regimen. This is especially true with adaptogenic herbs, as several of them interact with prescription medications and are not recommended for people with certain conditions.

PROFESSIONAL HELP: If none of these natural remedies alleviate your feelings, it may be time to talk to a professional. Licensed therapists can evaluate your case and provide counseling services to help you develop plans to correct problem areas in your life.

IMPORTANT NOTE ON EXERCISE: Being physically active has been proven to help prevent and alleviate the symptoms of stress, depression, and anxiety. What you may not know is that recent research[xxi] shows that if you are chronically stressed, it may not be a good idea to engage in high intensity forms of exercise as your body's ability to repair and respond to *acute* stress — such as exercise — is hindered because its resources are essentially used up. If you feel that your brain is tired, the rest of your body may be tired as well, which is why it may not be a great idea to engage in a strenuous activity.

Instead of going for a high intensity interval training class, cardio, or a bootcamp, try to balance your energy with a more calming, soothing way to move your body. Just like with everything else in this book, it's all about balance. One of my favorite things to do when I am stressed out is yoga and/or Pilates as they combine physical poses, controlled breathing, and meditation or relaxation. Yoga not only contributes to reduced stress, but also helps lower your blood pressure and heart rate.

BOTTOM LINE: Stress is an inevitable part of life. A little bit of short-term stress may be quite helpful in certain situations, but stress that goes beyond the short term can get you in trouble. You can improve the way you respond to stress: first by realizing what stressors you have; then by finding ways to avoid or change some of the situations that create negative stress. There are other techniques that you can use to relax your body, mind, and emotional levels.

CHECK-IN QUESTIONS

How were your energy levels on a scale of 1 to 10?

Did you feel fatigued or sluggish?

Can you think clearly?

Did you feel tired?

Did you feel bloated?

Did you have headaches? (If yes, how many?)

Did you go to the bathroom regularly?

Is your skin clear?

Did you have cravings?

Did you binge?

Did you eat or snack compulsively or mindlessly?

Is your sleep regular?

Did you have trouble concentrating or brain fog?

Did you suffer with mood swings?

Did you ever feel anxious, fearful, or nervous?

Did you feel physically weak?

Did you get sick?

Did you have bad breath?

Did you have heartburn?

Did you have stomach or intestinal pain?

Did you experience ringing in your ears?

Did you feel the need to urinate urgently or frequently?

Did you have pain or aches in your muscles and joints?

Did you feel stiff or limited in your movements?

"Does refusing to go to the gym count as resistance training?"

WEEK 11

THE RIGHT WORKOUT FOR YOU

Did you know that three-quarters of Americans and 37% of the UK population *never* exercise in their life or play a sport? Being sedentary is one of the core problems of our modern lifestyle. Along with eating a balanced, wholesome diet, we need to exercise regularly in order to experience true health.

You have probably heard countless times how exercise is 'good for you', but if you're like most Americans, you just don't do it. It's not that you don't want to, but with all the pressures of work, friends, and family, it's hard to find the strength, the time, and the willpower.

But did you know that if you start moving your body on a regular basis you will reduce cravings, regulate your appetite, improve your overall metabolism, reduce cortisol levels (the stress hormone that promotes belly fat), reduce inflammation, and get better sleep? Besides, working out helps your body function properly and aids with the detox process.

For me, the real problem with working out has always been that I have approached it as a way to change my body and not because I wanted to feel good. The good news: it doesn't have to be that way! It was only a few years into my healing journey, after many attempts to work out consistently that I was finally able to shift my mindset around it and it has truly been life changing.

To step you closer to doing the same, let's take a look at my shifts:

Undercommit to overachieve: The first (and biggest) step for me to get consistent with my workouts was to learn to not overcommit. This can sound completely counterintuitive at first, but I have a really good reason. Let me explain. The concept is a bit the same as dieting: If I tell you to not eat something, you want it more; but if I tell you that you can have whatever you want, you will be more likely to make better choices.

Here is how that works with exercising. The majority of influencers, doctors, and programs out there want you to train five times a week (if not seven)! I mean, that's just bull*hit for a start! Life happens. Some days you are tired, some you are too busy. And guess what happens if you skip one workout? You feel awful about yourself! Before you know it, you've skipped a couple of days in a row, then it'll be a week, a month... And here you are again with your yo-yo workout routine.

Here's how to not fall for that anymore: Commit to working out one time a week. That's right, just once a week, making sure you don't skip it. Pay attention to how good you feel afterwards and let that be your drive and motivation.

Now, here's what happens. Some weeks, you *will* only go and train once. But other weeks, you will have more energy and go twice or even three times. All you have to do is make that one day your non-negotiable. Before you know it, maybe in a few months' time, that one day will have become an automatic habit and your body will crave more.

Make it fun: Some people enjoy going with a partner. Personally, I like to fly solo as it gives me more freedom and flexibility.

The rule here is to find something you actually enjoy. Don't sign up for the gym just to do something when you find it boring to lift weights. You will not be consistent that way. Look for a gym or studio close to your house that offers different classes and try new stuff until you find something that speaks to you. It's when you find something you love and look forward to that you'll be more likely to stick with it. For example, I *hate the gym* and lifting weights. On the other hand, I *love music and movement*. I know I will push myself more if I have people around me doing the same exercises, so for me classes are the perfect combo.

Variety is key: I love switching things up, which is why I am obsessed with ClassPass, a monthly subscription that allows me to try different studios and activities in all the major cities around the world! If you don't have ClassPass in your area, I suggest signing up to a gym that has a mix of classes. I never do the same workout two days in a row (also because, most of the time, I only work out two or three times a week, as I always have a rest day in between). If you want to join and get a £40 discount, you can use my invite code: http://class.ps/mrPPU

Listen to your body: This was a true game-changer! We already covered this a little bit in Week 10 when talking about stress, but here's the thing: you have to *listen to your body*. If you are tired, don't go for a strenuous workout. Find something soothing. If you had a great day or woke up full of energy, then pick something to keep that energy up. You have to learn to be in flow and that is only done by balancing the energy you have inside and asking yourself how you're feeling before engaging in an activity. Are you tired? Go for a walk. Are you happy? A class with music is great. You get the idea.

Your new goal should be to work out once a week and try to move your body for at least 30 minutes, preferably every day of the week to keep your body strong and healthy. Here are some examples of how to do it:

- Get off the subway or bus one stop earlier

- Take the stairs instead of the elevator

- Go on nightly jogs or walk with a friend or your dog

- Take a brisk daily walk around the block during your lunch hour

- Ride your bike to work

- Park a couple of blocks away from work

- Play your favorite sport

Anything that will involve you moving your body counts, so get creative. Try new classes, get outdoors, play with your children or your dog in the park, or combine different sports.

REMEMBER: What we are trying to do here is build the foundation for a new lifestyle that you can carry with you forever, not another quick fix you will drop in a few months. So, don't overcommit (like trying to fit in a workout daily) or choose crazy workouts that you don't like — or even hate! —

just to get quick results. Doing this could have the opposite effect, as strenuous workouts can bring more stress to your body and cause you to gain weight. It also increases the risk of injuries. It's all about finding what works for you.

TRY: FIND YOUR DOSHA WEEK

One way to find what works for you is by discovering your Ayurvedic type or your dosha, which can tell you a lot about what suits your body composition… and what doesn't! Discovering my dosha was a complete game-changer for the way I look at exercise. Choosing exercise that is right for your dosha can be helpful in bringing balance to your body and mind. But let's take it a step back: what is a dosha?

Ayurveda is an ancient school of medicine from India, which, like Traditional Chinese Medicine, sees human health as a whole: mind, body, and spirit. Every person can be described as one of the three doshas: vata, pitta, or kapha. Doshas are the energies that make up every individual and that perform different physiological functions in the body:

1. Vata: The energy that controls bodily functions associated with motion, including blood circulation, breathing, blinking, and your heartbeat.

- In balance: There is creativity and vitality.

- Out of balance: Can produce fear and anxiety.

2. Pitta: The energy that controls the body's metabolic systems, including digestion, absorption, nutrition, and your body's temperature.

- In balance: Leads to contentment and intelligence.

- Out of balance: Can cause ulcers and anger.

3. Kapha: The energy that controls growth in the body. It supplies water to all body parts, moisturizes the skin, and maintains the immune system.

- In balance: Expressed as love and forgiveness.

- Out of balance: Can lead to insecurity and envy.

Each person has all three doshas within, but usually one or two dominate. Dosha proportions determine your physiological and personality traits, as well as general likes and dislikes. Here is a simplified rundown of each type:

Vata-predominant types: These people are creative, quick learners, and easily grasp new knowledge, but they also forget quickly. Body-wise they are slender and tall. They walk fast, usually have cold hands and feet, and feel discomfort in cold climates. Generally, they have dry skin and hair, and don't perspire much. Excitable, lively, fun personality, vata types change moods often. They have a hard time with daily routines, act on impulse, and often have racing, disjointed thoughts. With high energy in short bursts, they have a tendency to tire easily and to overexert. Full of joy and enthusiasm when in balance, when out of balance, they respond to stress with fear, worry, and anxiety.

Pitta-predominant types: They are sharp-minded, orderly, and focused, with good concentration powers. When in balance, they are assertive, self-confident, and entrepreneurial, but when out of balance they become aggressive, demanding, pushy. They are competitive by nature and enjoy challenges.

They usually have strong digestion and a good appetite. They get irritated if they miss or have to wait for a meal. Body-wise, their skin is fair or reddish, often with freckles. They burn easily in the sun and are uncomfortable in sunny or hot weather, as heat makes them tired. They perspire a lot. Usually with a medium physique, strong, and well-built. Their typical physical problems include rashes or inflammations of the skin, acne, boils, skin cancer, ulcers, heartburn, acid stomach, insomnia, dryness, or burning.

When under stress, pittas become irritated and angry but are usually passionate and romantic. They are good public speakers with generally good management and leadership ability but can become authoritarian. They are also subject to temper tantrums, impatience, and anger.

Kapha-predominant types: Easygoing, relaxed, and slow-paced, kaphas are affectionate, loving, forgiving, compassionate, and non-judgmental in nature. They are usually stable, reliable, and faithful. Physically, they are strong and with a sturdy, heavier build, but they have the most energy of all constitutions. With soft hair and skin, they also have the tendency to have large 'soft' eyes and a low, soft voice. They also tend toward being overweight and may suffer from sluggish digestion. Kapha don't like cold, damp weather. Physical problems include colds and congestion, sinus headaches, respiratory problems including asthma, allergies, and atherosclerosis (hardening of the arteries).

Usually, they are slow speakers, reflecting a deliberate thought process. They are slower learners but have an outstanding long-term memory. More self-sufficient and gentle, kaphas essentially have an undemanding approach to life. With excellent health and a good immune system, they strive to maintain harmony and peace in their surroundings.

They can be prone to depression and tend to be possessive and hold on to things.

Pretty interesting, no?! But why am I bringing this up? Because discovering my doshas and choosing a workout routine compatible with my dosha type has drastically transformed the way I perceive exercise. Working out went from a struggle to a true pleasure and something I look forward to.

Curious to discover your Dosha? You can ***take the test here*** below by answering the following questions:

Which most accurately describes your body?
- a) Naturally thin, lanky, slender
- b) Medium Built, good muscular build
- c) Curvy, bigger built

How easily do you gain weight?
- a) Next to impossible; have to remember to eat to try not to lose weight
- b) Moderately; can lose or gain weight if I really try and can put on muscle easily
- c) Too easily; put on weight just by looking at food and have a hard time losing it

What are your eyes like?
- a) On the smaller side and actively moving
- b) Have a penetrating deep gaze
- c) Big and beautiful

What is your skin like?
- a) Tends to get dry, quite thin, has visible veins
- b) Oily, acne prone, has a reddish tint
- c) Moist, smooth, thick, combination

What is your hair like?
  a) Dry, Freezy, prone to split ends and breakage
  b) Fine, oily, tendency towards thinning and/or graying
  c) Thick, abundant, more on the oily side

What are your joints like?
  a) Prominent, tend to crack, often aching, injury prone
  b) Flexible, Agile
  c) Large, well padded

What is your digestion like?
  a) Variable: sometimes good, sometimes bad
  b) Strong and powerful
  c) Slow and weak

What is your elimination like?
  a) Tends towards constipation
  b) Regular, tends towards loose stool
  c) Thick, long, sluggish

Which digestive imbalances do you feel more?
  a) Bloating and gas
  b) Heartburn acidic stomach
  c) Heaviness after eating and water retention

How is your body temperature?
  a) Always cold; prefer hot weather
  b) Usually warm; prefer cold weather
  c) Pretty adaptable; I don't like cold wet weather though

What is your temperament like?
  a) Enthusiastic, vivacious and creative
  b) Driven, passionate, ambitious
  c) Easy-going, giving, patient

What are your negative traits?
  a) Anxious, fearful, and or nervous
  b) Competitive, aggressive and or impatient
  c) Lonely, depressed, and or jealous

How do you sleep?
  a) Difficulty falling asleep, wake up often
  b) Moderate and sound
  c) Deep and long

How is your memory?
  a) Quick to remember, quick to forget
  b) Medium but accurate with facts
  c) Hard time remembering but then sustained

How are you with money and material possessions?
  a) Impulsive shopper; buy things and forget about them
  b) Calculate at shopper; spend on luxuries that are worth it
  c) Hoarder; have a hard time letting things go

What subject are you most drawn to words?
  a) The arts, spirituality, philosophy, literature, big picture stuff
  b) Business, science, law, engineering, calculate it stuff
  c) Counseling, teaching, human resources, and care giving, hands on stuff

Now count how many A, B, and C answer you got. A answers represent Vata. B answers represents Pitta. C answers represents Kapha. The Dosha with your highest number is your primary Dosha. The second highest-number is your secondary Dosha and the Dosha with the lowest number is your tertiary.

Once you discover your dosha, here are the workouts that may fit you best:

Vata exercises: Those who are predominantly vata benefit enormously from **grounding exercises** such as yoga, easy walking, cycling, weightlifting, Pilates, and dance. Vata types have bursts of energy but tend to tire quickly. Feeling dizzy, exhausted, or on the verge of cramping are all signs of overdoing it. In the winter, vata need to work out indoors.

Pitta exercises: Pitta has a strong drive and tends to like *challenging sports* such as skiing, hiking, tennis, and mountain-climbing. Swimming is an ideal exercise for pitta dosha, because the water cools the heat of pitta and relieves the accumulated tension of the day. Other calming and relaxing physical exercises are yoga, leisurely walks outdoors in a beautiful area, rollerblading, and Pilates.

Kapha exercises: Kapha dosha have strong, steady energy and great physical strength. Therefore, *cardiovascular exercises* and endurance sports are the way to go. Some examples are: long-distance running, aerobics, dance, soccer, rowing, and so on. If you are predominantly kapha, your biggest challenge may be finding the motivation to exercise. If you have not been exercising for a while, you can break the inertia by starting with brisk walking, beginning with half an hour.

BOTTOM LINE: Exercising is the best antidepressant and antianxiety treatment you can get. It has tons of health benefits for your mind and body. As long as you pick something you enjoy, it will improve energy, well-being, and self-esteem. Take those 30 minutes a day as a treat to yourself and move your body in a way that makes you feel happy and excited. Don't sign up for a strenuous bootcamp or crossfit class that you hate just to get quick results. The only way you will ever stick to an exercise plan is if you enjoy what you are doing. If you are pushing yourself to follow a workout program for the sake of your health or to change your body but aren't enjoying it, you are unlikely to stick with it.

Choosing exercises suited to your mind-body type will give you the greatest benefits and enjoyment. Discovering my dosha has helped me tremendously and should help you too. Experiment with new workouts and bring variety to your routine.

"Don't work out to change your body; work out to feel better and your body will change as a result." – Eleonora C. Bastos

DON'T FORGET: TRAIN YOUR MIND

Just as important as training your body is keeping your mind active. We know that the human brain is a powerful organ, but many of us aren't aware of how much *more* powerful it can become through deliberate training. Lots of studies have linked meditation with both physical and mental health benefits, from reduced depression and anxiety to improved immune system functioning. Boost brainpower by spending time thinking positively, meditating, reading, or practicing activities that require thinking. Sudoku, Memory, and Chess are great examples of games that also can boost your brain activity.

CHECK-IN QUESTIONS

Did you feel fatigued or sluggish?

Can you think clearly?

Did you feel tired?

Did you feel bloated?

Did you have headaches? (If yes, how many?)

Did you go to the bathroom regularly?

Is your skin clear?

Did you have cravings?

Did you binge?

Did you eat or snack compulsively or mindlessly?

Is your sleep regular?

Did you have trouble concentrating or brain fog?

Did you suffer with mood swings?

Did you ever feel anxious, fearful, or nervous?

Did you feel physically weak?

Did you get sick?

Did you have bad breath?

Did you have heartburn?

Did you have stomach or intestinal pain?

Did you experience ringing in your ears?

Did you feel the need to urinate urgently or frequently?

Did you have pain or aches in your muscles and joints?

Did you feel stiff or limited in your movements?

"I am on a seefood diet. I see food and I eat it."

WEEK 12

HOW TO HAVE A LIFE AND STILL BE HEALTHY

As I was growing up, I remember my mom saying, "A little bit of everything in moderation is never going to kill you." At the time, I restricted and controlled everything I ate, so I would disagree with her because of my fear of food. Now I can attest to her saying being true. Unless you suffer with a chronic condition, in which case you will need to be more conscious about your choices.

I like to go about my life from a place of choice where I am consciously **choosing what to eat** because I know how it impacts my body. With this book, I hope you are a little closer to understanding foods too and being able to make conscious choices.

Although Nutella, pizza, and pasta (my treats) should be avoided most of the time because of their health implications, sometimes they are "good for the soul" as my mom would also say.

The same goes for whatever makes you happy. A more relaxed approach to what you eat will get you far.

EATING AT A RESTAURANT

To me the worst part of any diet plan is limiting your choices, which makes it really hard to be able to socialize and enjoy life. Going out to eat should be a fun experience, not a stressful situation that makes you feel anxious or guilty! The goal of this book has been to set out the stepping-stones for a new lifestyle, sustainable for the rest of your life, shifting away from the regular dieting traps. So, if you go out for dinner once a week, *enjoy yourself!*

If you tend to go out more than once a week, here are a few tricks I use to stay healthy while enjoying dining out with friends, whether it's dinner at their place or out at a restaurant:

Have a healthy snack before you go: This is one of my all-time favorite tips and by far the most useful one of all! I know that this can sound weird but it's the same concept as not going shopping on an empty stomach. Get it? Eating something before going out will curb your appetite and prevent you from diving into the breadbasket when you sit down at the table or ordering every unhealthy item on the menu. I'm not suggesting eating a full meal before dinner, but a small healthy snack will have you making better choices. I usually have a half-serving of protein shake about 30 minutes before heading out the door, but you could also try carrot sticks and hummus, celery and peanut butter, a handful of nuts, or any other healthy snack you like. Trust me: game-changer!

Go prepared: If you know which restaurant you are going to, check the menu beforehand. This way you can familiarize yourself with what's served and get an idea of what you want. If you are very social with your friends and get together multiple times a week, ask the host what they are making and if you can bring something. If it's a not-so-healthy option, grab that healthy snack before heading over so you will eat a smaller portion or bring over a healthy side dish.

Avoid or limit drinks: If I go out more than once a week, I tend to order only one drink per night. By avoiding alcoholic drinks, your health and your wallet will thank you. Whenever you are entertaining clients or are out for business dinners, here is the game: drink one glass of water for every alcoholic drink. This means you can't order another drink until you've downed a full glass of water.

Ask for the dressing on the side: Dressing is always tricky when going out, as it's usually the unhealthiest part of your meal and restaurants tend to put too much of it on your food. Ask if you can have the dressing on the side so you are in charge of how much dressing goes on.

Make substitutions. Speak kindly to your server to see if you can replace the fries or fattening side dish with something lighter and healthier like veggies.

Keep it simple: If you are trying to eat healthily at a restaurant, typically the simpler the meal the better. Try to avoid food with cream, added sauces, or breadcrumb coatings, so you can avoid all the additives that usually come with them.

Avoid richer foods: On the whole, steer clear of 'au gratin', 'buttered', 'creamed/creamy', 'hollandaise', 'cheesy', 'fried' or 'rich' menu descriptions. All of these have a lot of added fat, cholesterol, and additives that are not worth your while. If you really cannot resist, limit the splurge to twice a month.

Be creative: Combine appetizers and sides to create a meal. Just because it says 'entrees' on the menu doesn't mean you have to order them that way. Portions sizes are out of control these days, so opting for a starter and a side can go a long way.

Just eat half: Especially if you go to restaurant chains, where portions are crazy, ask for a doggy bag. There is nothing wrong with that.

Make sure you like what you eat: I know this may sound silly but being present, savoring your meal, eating slowly, truly tasting your food and checking in with your own enjoyment can actually make you feel satisfied with less and help your digestion and nutrient absorption.

Last but not least, ***enjoy yourself!***

Use all these tips whenever possible but remember to enjoy your meal. You cannot control everything, so give yourself a break and take pleasure in some tasty food that's really worth your while. Remember, one bad meal will not undo your progress. Have a good time and don't allow this meal to be a source of anxiety.

SOCIAL EVENTS AND GATHERINGS

For the longest time, social gatherings have been paired with food and alcohol. And although it is true that one piece of cake or a pasta dinner will not sabotage your health, if you tend to have a busy social life, staying healthy can be a tricky business, especially at the beginning of your health journey.

A birthday on Tuesday, a business dinner on Thursday, a family event on Sunday... And then there's the gala event, the engagement party, the bridal shower, the catered mixer, the BBQ, the rugby game... I mean, you get it. Trying to stay healthy while syncing your social and professional event calendar could be like mixing oil and water — a frustrating effort.

The truth is that no one wants to feel restricted or like they're missing out on social opportunities. But here's the good news: You can still keep your health on track even with the busiest social calendar. How?

I know you've heard it a million times but failing to plan is planning to fail. What I mean by this is that if you have a game plan on how to navigate whatever social situation you're going to be in, nine times out of ten it will be possible for you to attend and enjoy your outing while 'being healthy'. And the times you can't, well then, just enjoy the s**t out of it!

Here are my best tips on how you can have your cake (and ice cream and burgers) and eat it too — without sacrificing your social life or health goals.

1. DO NOT ARRIVE AT THE EVENT HUNGRY

This is the Golden Rule, and by far the most useful tip! By eating something before going out, you will curb your appetite, which will prevent you from overindulging. Have that healthy snack before you leave or down a protein shake!

2. PLAN AHEAD

This is one of my sneakiest tricks after the Golden Rule. Planning ahead is great because it helps you feel good and enjoy yourself without feeling restricted. What I mean by *planning* is for you to ask your host what's on the menu, so you can offer to bring something healthy if there's nothing healthy planned and decide what to save space for. (My favorite!)

For me, this little trick allows me to enjoy myself without feeling restricted and it has become a natural part of planning any social occasion.

I always allow myself a treat for social gatherings and I call it 'something delicious'. This is something I choose to eat that's out of the norm for me. It's something I am really excited about and that I eat with zero (and I mean Z-E-R-O) guilt.

I even make sounds while chewing, closing my eyes, and plastering a big fat grin on my face. Here is the proof of the enjoyment.

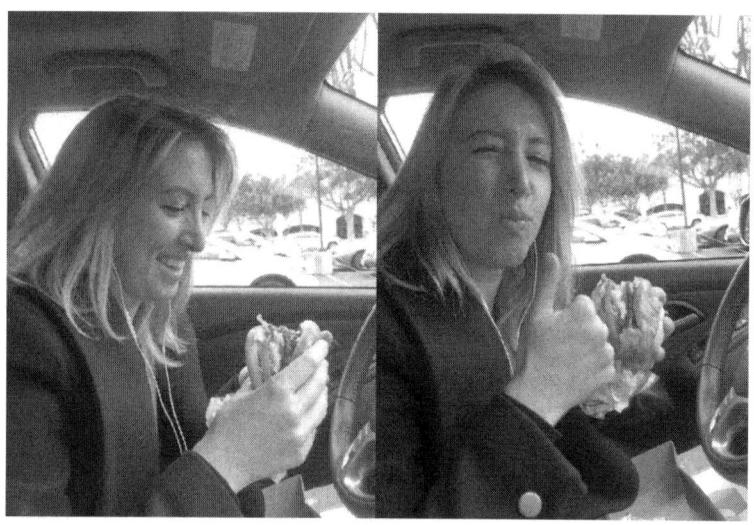

Planning ahead allows me to choose in advance what treat I intend to have, get excited about it, and then have something to look forward to the whole time. It can be a muffin, pizza, pasta, or a chocolate chip cookie. And the best part is that I get so excited about that treat that I don't ever feel like I'm missing out on anything else.

This works so well for events with a buffet. Scan the whole table first and choose your treat. Adjust the rest of your meal accordingly. Get it?

However, this works only when you learn to not feel guilty afterwards. Really and truly not guilty. The only way to do that is understanding that one not-so-great choice will not undo your progress.

3. AVOID MINDLESS EATING

One of the easiest things to do at social gatherings is to get carried away with eating all kinds of foods that you might not typically eat, just because they are there. When you first enter a room, take note of where the buffet table, bar, and dessert table are located. Place yourself as far away as possible. Sound silly? Maybe. But by standing near the buffet, people tend to eat mindlessly while chatting away, resulting in overeating.

4. CONTROL YOUR PORTIONS

The problem with an abundance of (delicious) food at your disposal is watching portions. I use a small plate, order a starter and share the main course or fill half the plate with veggies or salad (watching out for the dressing), leaving only half the plate available for the main. Also, before making a choice, scan the whole buffet or menu and 'pick your battle'.

5. EAT SLOWLY

Eat slowly, savor the food, and try to avoid having seconds immediately after you're done eating what's on your plate. Why? Remember it takes about 20 to 30 minutes for your body to register how much you ate. If you are still hungry after waiting 20 minutes, then go for more.

6. REMEMBER IT'S ABOUT NUTRIENT DENSITY

Don't count your calories! By now, I hope you know this. When choosing what goes on your plate, remember it's about nutrient density: keep half for veggies, quarter for proteins, and a quarter for carbs.

7. LIMIT ALCOHOL

Did you know that we generally eat more when we've had a few drinks? There have been a number of studies on the topic (the most recent one published in 2017 Nature Communications, looked at how ethanol alcohol affects the body, brain, and actions of mice). Not only does drinking alcohol do your overall health no good, but it also makes you overeat. Limit the amount of alcohol you consume (one glass of water for every alcoholic drink) and you'll not only save yourself form a hangover, but you'll be less likely to overindulge.

8. JUST RELAX

Try to eat healthily and move your body most of the week, but don't forget that you're human! You are not meant to be perfect. It's okay to enjoy yourself, have a glass of wine, a dance, and a chat. Just do so in moderation and you'll feel confident, in control, and positive. Enjoy!

MEAL REPLACEMENTS AND PROTEIN BARS

Okay, let's be clear here. *I do not advocate replacing your meals with meal substitutes as a way of living.* In fact, the whole notion of calories in/calories out and replacing meals with shakes to lose weight is what got me into the endless cycle of dieting, disordered eating, and created a very unhealthy relationship with food.

This could be quite a shocker to read for people who know me and my family, because I come from a family that advocates the opposite and made an exceptional living out of this belief.

That said, sometimes having a *simple, clean protein powder* on hand when you are busy running around or adding it to your morning smoothie instead of having a proper breakfast makes life easy while keeping you well-nourished. Occasionally, for those reasons, I use meal replacement powders and protein bars to supplement my diet at breakfast, when I don't have time to stop for lunch or when I need to boost my stamina in the afternoon so I can make it through to dinner. Yes, it happens and it's fine.

Why don't I tell you about them sooner? Because, as I explained, whole foods are *way better* and I believe everyone should understand how a balanced diet (low in toxins and high in nutrition) works. This book was designed to help you release your reliance on unnatural, processed foods (at least for a few weeks). If I had told you this at the beginning, you might have resorted to this first, which is not great. I'll tell you why.

Meal replacements and protein bars are **still processed**. Most manufacturers don't make good products, but market them just right, which creates lots of confusion (and inflammation) in those buying them. In fact, manufacturers usually pack these products with sugar, or worse, sugar substitutes, chemicals, fillers, the list goes on. Always read the label before buying something. If you need a refresher on how to understand labels, go to the Week 3 chapter. And always remember that meal replacements and protein bars are not the same as a good meal — but they're quick and easy, and certainly can make a good snack.

ALCOHOL: SHOULD YOU PUT THAT DRINK DOWN?

I'm not here to lecture you about your current alcohol consumption habits, but like with everything else, balance is key. There is nothing wrong with enjoying a boozy night out with your friends once in a while. I love a glass of wine or two on occasion. I'm Italian, what do you expect?!

But if you're drinking to boost your confidence, repress emotions like stress or sadness, or you are a daily drinker, you may want to consider a different approach for those feelings. In fact, overconsumption of alcohol could get you into trouble. Here are a few reasons you may want to ease up on drinking:

It encourages your body to burn 36% less fat, which means you will store more fat when you eat.

Alcohol depletes vital nutrients including B vitamins, which can result in anxiousness, tiredness, and depression.

Mixers are mostly made by sugar and chemical additives. We already saw what these do to your health.

Liver: Excessive alcohol strains the liver. A distressed **liver** can lead to dry, itchy redness, acne, and dull and sagging skin. Heavy drinking takes a toll on the liver, and can lead to a variety of problems and liver inflammations including:

- Steatosis or fatty liver

- Alcoholic hepatitis

- Fibrosis

- Cirrhosis

Brain: Alcohol interferes with the brain's communication pathways and can affect the way the brain works. These disruptions can change mood and behavior and make it harder to think clearly and move with coordination.

Immune system: Drinking too much can weaken your immune system, making your body a much easier target for disease. Chronic drinkers are more liable to contract diseases like pneumonia and tuberculosis than people who do not drink much. Also, drinking a lot on a single occasion slows your body's ability to ward off infections up to 24 hours after getting drunk.

Cancer: Drinking too much alcohol can increase your risk of developing certain cancers, including mouth, esophagus, throat, liver, and breast cancers.

Pancreas: Alcohol causes the pancreas to produce toxic substances that can eventually lead to pancreatitis, a dangerous inflammation and swelling of the blood vessels in the pancreas that prevents proper digestion.

Blood sugar: Alcohol creates mayhem with our blood glucose levels, which can result in cravings. It also impairs your impulse control, so you're more likely to eat greater quantities and to do so mindlessly.

Digestive system: It provokes a leaky gut, candida, and inflames your liver.

Weight gain: If you have one glass of wine a day, over the course of a year, it can add up to eleven pounds of weight gain.

Sleep: It disrupts your sleep and increases depression.

Now, it's entirely up to you whether or not you want to cut alcohol from your life completely. If you still want to be a responsible social drinker, here are a few tips to minimize the harmful effects of alcohol:

Try to avoid ciders and sweet wines. Besides getting a horrible hangover, they are loaded with sugar, which can result in irritability, mood swings, and weight gain.

Skip the flavored liqueurs, sugary mixers, and soda mixers. Instead, try to have your liqueur on the rocks or mix it with water, sparkling water, lime, or orange juice.

Avoid drinking when you are eating. When you eat and drink at the same time, your body's top priority is to metabolize alcohol first and then break down the food. This will cause weight gain, gas, bloating, and other digestive discomforts.

The morning after, reach for coconut water when you wake up. Coconut water is naturally rich in electrolytes — one serving offers 569mg of potassium — which makes it incredibly hydrating. An added bonus: coconut water has more flavor than regular H_2O, which may make it easier to stomach.

Eat some liver-loving ingredients. Turmeric, cinnamon, kale, broccoli, beetroot, avocado, and lemon are all fantastic foods for helping support the liver, so eat plenty of these during the day before you go out.

Having a green juice will do wonders for your body. Alcohol dehydrates you and robs your body of electrolytes and nutrients, which is the reason you feel not-so-great the morning after. If you don't feel like having a green juice before you drink, make sure to do as soon you wake up in the morning!

One glass of alcohol, one glass of water. This simple trick has saved me so many times! Make it a point to drink a glass of water for every glass of alcohol you have. It won't kill your buzz, but it will definitely save you in the morning. In fact, one of the main reasons why you feel so bad the morning after is because of dehydration. Simply sipping some water in between your drinks will help your body replenish the water it loses, and you will recover faster.

BOTTOM LINE: Alcohol can be a medicine or a poison. When consumed in small quantities, alcohol — even hard liqueur — offers antioxidant protection. Red wine is especially healthful. So much has been written about the health-boosting benefits of resveratrol, which protects the brain, improves insulin resistance, and fights both heart disease and cancer. However, when alcohol is tossed back in large doses, it is poison to the body as we saw here.

How much alcohol is too much? Try to limit your alcohol intake to a couple of times a week, but if it's a daily habit, consume no more than one drink a day while you wean yourself down to twice a week. Remember, moderation is key.

When you eliminate alcohol, you may feel better in a few weeks and you will help your body change the flora in your gut, which is critical for keeping you healthy!

GET TO THE ROOT OF IT: (DYS)FUNCTIONAL WESTERN MEDICINE

We live in an amazing society, where every possible answer is at our fingertips. In fact, with a simple smartphone, tablet, or computer, we have access in seconds to the world's biggest encyclopedia: Google. Nowadays, you can Google absolutely anything and get an answer instantly, so it's time to start using this tool to your advantage and transforming yourself into a health detective for your own health.

What I would like you to do is to **start shifting your perspective** on illness and health challenges. From a simple cold to more serious situations like autoimmune disease, cancer, and so forth, let go of the paradigm of functional Western medicine and investigate Eastern medicine approaches. Why? Because unfortunately there are many limitations with Western medicine:

- In most cases, Western medicine focuses on **curing the symptoms of the disease, rather than finding the cause** or root problem. This can lead you to need a lifetime for drug therapy. The sad part is that most of the time this happens for monetary reasons, to make sure you keep on buying medications for as long as possible. How do you think the pharmaceutical industry is worth 300 billion a year[xxii]?

- ***Pharmaceutical drugs have sides effects*** and sometimes this is a downward spiral where you find yourself in a cycle of taking drugs to deal with the unwanted effects of another drug, the one you were originally prescribed.

- Doctors are trained to give the ***same treatment to everyone*** with certain symptoms but have almost no knowledge on how to prevent you getting ill in the first place.

Don't get me wrong, doctors are great in emergency situations like if you break a leg, are in a car crash, or if you are seriously ill and need surgery. But as explained here, there are certain limitations that you cannot ignore. I am not saying that you should never see a doctor again or that you should stop listening to them. I would never suggest that. Indeed, I advise you to always check in with your health practitioner before making any changes, especially if you are critically ill or currently on medication. But I encourage you to not just blindly put your health in the hands of whatever doctor fate and your health insurance happened to assign you, especially if you leave your doctor's office with a knot in your stomach, thinking you didn't really get the answers you needed.

That's where becoming your own investigator comes in. Always ask your doctor for ***the cause of your condition***. If they don't know what caused your symptoms, do some research and work to fix the root of the problem.

TRY IT OUT: Next time you have something wrong with your body, like a headache, search a term like 'what ***causes*** headaches' rather than taking a pill to kill the ***symptom***. Some sources of information that I trust are: Medical News

Today, Dr. Axe and Dr. Mercola, MayoClinic, Health Line, and Harvard Health.

This applies to everything that goes wrong with your body, from simple flu to more severe cases like chronic diseases: think about the root cause. If you cannot find the exact answer for what your body is going through, consult a naturopath, a holistic practitioner (like myself), or an Eastern medicine doctor, but please don't just settle. It is your responsibility to be healthy and proactive in looking for alternatives.

NOW IS THE TIME

Last, but not least, let's address smoking. If you don't have a habit, you're one of the lucky ones and can skip this section. And if you do? I'm not here to tell you why you should quit smoking because you are not stupid. You know exactly why smoking is bad for you. However, I am here to share my experience with you and tell you what worked for me.

As an ex-smoker, I know that I was only able to quit once I felt healthy in my body. Only when I didn't have to think about healthy eating or consistent workouts any more was I ready to quit. At that time, I tried not to smoke for 21 days. And it was amazing! What a change it made in my performance. That's when I decided to quit for good. I went from almost two packets a day to smoking socially to quitting completely. I just don't have the need for it anymore.

By now, if you have been following this book as it was intended, your diet will be healthier, your cravings and sugar addiction will be all but gone, and you may well have seen a great increase in your energy and focus. All of this will make the battle to quit smoking much less of a battle. So, if you ever wanted to quit, now is the time!

Of all the quit smoking programs I've seen offered through the wellness work I do, Allen Carr's Easy Way is by far the best at getting results. I've seen people with zero desire to quit, quit after one seminar. Incredible!

That said, there are many different ways to quit, so I recommend you do your research and try what you believe will work for you.

Whatever you choose, ***don't make the mistake of resorting to pharmaceutical 'quit-smoking drugs'*** like Chantix, Zyban, Wellbutrin, vaporizers, or others. Like all drugs, they come with a wide spectrum of side effects that are harmful to your health. The types of drugs listed above in particular also carry much higher risks of depression, violence, and even suicide. So please, do yourself a favor and ***steer well clear***.

SELF-CARE

In this high-paced society where so much is asked of us all the time, it's easy to forget to take care of our personal needs. A few years ago, I read this quote that has stuck with me ever since: "You can't pour from an empty cup." In order to perform properly and take care of others, we have to take care of ourselves first.

Self-care has become a bit of a buzzword lately, but I often feel it is poorly understood by most people. Perhaps you keep seeing it mentioned in self-help books or magazine articles, yet don't have a clear sense of how you're supposed to add it to your life. So, what exactly is self-care?

As indulgent as it may sound, self-care is a broad term that incorporates just about anything you do to feel good, not only in your body, but also to feel happy, healthy, and at peace in your mind. It can come in many different forms and there's no manual or one-size-fits-all approach to it.

TOP FIVE BENEFITS OF SELF-CARE

Taking a few hours for some much-deserved self-care is an effective way to manage stress. The top benefits of self-care are:

- **Better productivity.** When you learn how to say no to things that over-extend you and start making time for things that matter more, you slow life down in a wonderful way. This brings your goals into sharper focus and helps you concentrate on what you're doing.

- **Improved resistance to disease.** There is evidence that most self-care activities activate your parasympathetic nervous system (PNS). What this means is that your body goes into a restful, rejuvenating mode, helping fortify the immune system. With better self-care often comes fewer colds, cases of flu, and upset stomachs.

- **Enhanced self-esteem.** When you regularly carve out time that's only about being good to yourself and meeting your own needs, you send a positive message to your subconscious. Specifically, you treat yourself like you matter and have intrinsic value. This can go a long way toward discouraging negative self-talk, your critical inner voice.

- **Increased self-knowledge.** Practicing self-care requires thinking about what you really love to do. The exercise of figuring out what makes you feel passionate and inspired can help you understand yourself a lot better. Sometimes, this can even spark a change in career or a reprioritization of previously abandoned hobbies.

- **More to give.** When you're good to yourself, you might think you're being selfish but, in reality, it allows you to be more compassionate to others. Remember, you can't pour from an empty cup.

BURNOUT: WHEN SELF-CARE BECOMES SELF-SABOTAGE

In an ideal world, we would all be able to carve out enough time to go leisurely about our day, pausing for 20 minutes here and there to meditate or take a walk, end our day with an hour-long yoga class or workout, and come home to a nice warm bath followed by an amazing home cooked meal.

But let's be honest here… Reality is quite different.

Truth is that you are likely overwhelmed, tired, and stressed. You have a substantial commute to work, long and draining work hours, your home chores piling up, and your calendar is packed with social and extracurricular activities. We all know how important it is to do what makes us feel alive, nurtured, and well taken care of, but there are only so many hours in the day.

The central issue leading to burnout is that we keep ourselves too busy. So, is it possible that your self-care rituals are adding to that and becoming too much to the point of burnout?

The answer is yes!

Any busy professional who is committed to adding in self-care to their daily lives goes through this. Don't get me wrong. I'm a **huge believer in self-care rituals** and talk about their importance all the time with clients and in speaking engagements. However, oftentimes, I think introducing more self-care rituals and practices to an already busy schedule is just adding fuel to the fire.

It's not self-care if you're making that early morning gym session but then falling asleep on the bus to work or feeling exhausted the whole day. It's not self-care if you make it to your hair appointment but skip lunch. You get the picture.

When it comes to self-care, it's important to know what works for you. When self-care practices start to feel like a chore, that's a sign you have taken on too much under the guise of self-love and aren't fully able to commit to them or absorb their benefits. It's time to take a good, hard look at your current reality.

It's easy to forget that looking after your mental health isn't about being perfect. Good mental health isn't having a life planned down to the minute with vegan meals, exercise, meditation, coaching, yoga classes, long runs, and time with friends. Self-care is as much about the things you don't do as the things you do! Sometimes self-care is staying in bed. Sometimes it's cancelling that exercise after work to go straight home to the comfort of your PJs. Or otherwise it's skipping the morning workout and hitting snooze on the alarm. Sometime self-care is about saying no to invitations when you're simply too tired to enjoy them.

Remember this when you are thinking about your self-care routine; it's quality over quantity. It's not how many things you can fit into your day, but how those things make you feel inside. Follow your instinct and listen to your body. It is always talking to you.

BOTTOM LINE: Self-care is the act and attitude you take to maintain a standard of wellbeing, health, and personal happiness. It's what you do to add richness to your life, to make yourself feel full, nurtured, and taken care of. It can look different to different people, so you need to find what works for you! If you feel like your self-care routine is becoming a chore and adding more stress than nurturing and love, reassess what you are doing and remove anything that feels more like a burden. Invest more into what you want to keep.

Just remember that self-care is as much about what you don't do as what you do!

TRY: SELF-CARE STRATEGIES WEEK

There are several different ways to focus on self-care, many of which involve making time to get enough sleep, prioritizing healthy meals, ensuring a work-life balance with your schedule, and making time for friends. A simple but often overlooked form of self-care is having a self-pampering experience on a regular basis in your own home. As we said, whatever you choose to do, it needs to make you feel good physically and emotionally. Here are some of my favorite self-care practices, which I have divided into physical and emotional for convenience.

PHYSICAL SELF-CARE

- **Take a bath:** I love my bubble bath. I have one every Sunday night with my man! Get out the bubbles, essential oils and candles, and soak until you're wrinkled. Taking a bath with your partner creates an even more magical healing time to connect and reset your system.

- **Have a little spa night at home:** Personally, I love to combine my bath time with a little spa moment. Whether you have a tub or not, you can still have a spa night where you deep-condition your hair, use a replenishing face mask, shave, tend to your nails, and nourish your skin with a beautiful moisturizer. You must try it!

- **Get a massage:** This one is another of my favorites! If your budget doesn't allow for regular monthly massages with a professional, see if you can trade with a friend or your spouse, or use an electric massager.

- **Cuddle up:** Dive under a soft blanket while watching a movie or reading a book and drinking some warm tea.

- **Listen to music:** You can even burn candles, drink tea, and read a great book, or simply lie down to listen to the music with your eyes closed.

- **Sit outdoors:** Spend time in the heat of the afternoon sun staring at the sky and listening to some music.

- **Nap when you need it:** Just 20 minutes can make you feel mentally and physically refreshed.

- **Walk outdoors:** Focus on the beauty around you. What do you like of what you see?

- **Have a dance party in your house:** Put on your favorite tunes and dance around the house to your favorite songs. (This is my morning ritual!)

- **Hold your pet:** Pick up your pet and hold in your arms or snuggle up while listening to nice relaxing music.

- **Make a nice home cooked meal:** Maybe even try a new recipe.

- **Join a class.**

- **Learn a new sport.**

- **Set time aside to move your body daily.**

- **Go for a run or a walk:** Take your dog or go with a friend and leave the phone at home.

In addition to pampering yourself, more substantial forms of self-care involve healthy lifestyle choices like consuming a healthy diet, getting regular exercise, and being sure you get enough sleep.

EMOTIONAL AND SPIRITUAL SELF-CARE

- **Deliberately encourage yourself to laugh:** Especially at old memories or funny videos.

- **Take time to just sit with your thoughts and see what comes up:** You can call this meditation, but it does not have to be on a cushion with your legs crossed and eyes closed. I love doing this once a day with warm tea and relaxing instrumental music. I stare at the ceiling for 5 to 10 minutes. Just make sure to not be distracted.

- **See a therapist:** Even if it's just for 8 to 10 sessions of general personal development.

- **Make time to be with a friend or family member:** Make it someone who truly understands you, and makes you feel happy and at peace.

- **Let yourself cry when you need to.**

- **Be creative:** Whether through art, music, writing, or something else entirely.

- **Go on a trip:** Travel with the sole purpose of photographing things that inspire you.

SOCIAL SELF-CARE

- **Make a date:** Have lunch or dinner with your best friend.

- **Write an email:** Choose someone who lives far away, but who you miss.

- **Get back in touch:** Reach out to someone you like but haven't seen in a while.

- **Find like-minded people:** Consider joining a group of people who share your interests.

- **Quit the energy-draining situations:** Stop socializing with those who undermine or disempower you.

- **Strike up a conversation with someone interesting.**

- **Join a support group** for people who struggle with the same things you do.

- **Learn something:** Sign up for a class to learn something and meet new people at the same time.

BOTTOM LINE: Make a list of 5 to 10 things that make you feel alive, then ask yourself how you can better incorporate these into your life. Once you've decided it's time to start nurturing yourself and your body, be sure to block off some time for it where you won't be interrupted.

*"The best project
you will
ever work on
is YOU."*

THE END!

Our journey together in this book has come to an end.

You made it!

Over the last 12 weeks, you've done a lot for yourself. How do you feel about it? Well, I can tell you that I could not be prouder. I do hope you feel proud of yourself too.

If you have followed everything covered in this book, you should be experiencing wonderful improvements from the time you started. Take the time to review your progress, by re-reading the initial questionnaire. Where were you when you started? How are you feeling now? How did your energy level improve? Did you have less fatigue or fogginess? Did you lose weight? Did you feel less bloated? Did you look and feel better? Is your skin clear? Take a minute to write down all of your wins.

If you haven't gotten all the results you wanted, don't panic. Remember, this is just the beginning of a life-long journey. You have all the tools you need to continue being your own health detective and learning what works best for you.

Given the chance, your body will always heal itself, so you just need to give it what it needs in order to do its job. Your body is constantly talking to you by sending you signals; it's up to you to decode them and give your body what it needs.

Forget about restrictions, diets and calorie-counting, and focus on *nourishing your body* instead. Whenever you decide to eat something, analyze what nutrients you are putting in your body and adjust accordingly. One not-so-healthy choice every now and then will not harm you, so you can enjoy your favorite treats without feeling guilty.

Moderation is the key to maintaining your good health though, so try to be mindful about what you are feeding your body 90% of the time. The rest of the time? Just enjoy yourself!

And if you overdo it a bit, don't give up, don't stress out and don't starve yourself to 'make up for it'. Rather, just remember your long-term goal of feeling and looking your best. Then continue where you left off.

Lastly, don't forget that your mental and emotional state impacts how your body functions just as much as food does. It is imperative that you learn to address what you have inside and feed your soul with what it needs. You are the only person in charge of your own happiness, and nobody knows better than you what you like, want, and need to feel good. Find your passion, learn to say no, take time to rest, recharge, and enjoy life. You can't pour from an empty cup so make sure you do whatever it takes to feel happy and fulfilled.

Life is too short to live it feeling miserable in your body and mind. It's time for you to take charge. You deserve to be happy. You deserve to feel good in your skin. Seize responsibility for your own health and happiness and find your truth.

If I can do it, you can too.

Sending you love,

E.

BONUSES

HEALTHY SNACKS

Snacking is an effective way to fit extra nutrients into your diet, maintain a steady blood-sugar level while preventing overeating at mealtimes. Eating healthy snacks between meals becomes effective only if you are really hungry.

Eat any one of these snacks alone or pair two together.

- ½ cup cooked or raw veggies (carrots, broccoli, cucumber, celery, etc.)

- 1 apple, ¾ cup berries or ½ banana with 1 tbsp of peanut butter

- 1 handful of nuts or seeds. (Not more than once a day.)

- 2 tablespoons nut or seed butter and an apple

- 1 brown rice cake with hummus and celery. Sprinkle some salt and pepper on top for extra flavor.

- Celery sticks with no more of 2tbsp peanut butter

- 10 baby carrots with 2 tablespoons of hummus

- ¼ cup bean spread on 2 or 3 small crackers. Try Trader Joe's black bean dip, Desert Pepper's white bean or pinto bean spreads.

- 4 ounces plain coconut yogurt, plain almond yogurt or Greek yogurt

- ½ cup shelled edamame beans

- ½ cup shelled unsalted pistachios

- Crispy oven-baked falafels

- 2 hard boiled eggs

- 1 hard boiled egg and ½ avocado. (Dice everything, put oil, pepper and salt.)

- ½ avocado with 2 tbsp of cottage cheese

- 6 high-fiber, gluten-free crackers

- Wrap a slice of turkey around a quartered cucumber stick.

- Tuna salad with 4 or 5 small multi-grain crackers. (Mix up some tuna salad at the beginning of the week and use it for a quick high protein snack throughout the week. I love subbing Mayo with Vegenaise With multi-grain crackers, you have yourself a balanced snack.)

NATURAL REMEDIES

GASTRITIS/GERD

- **Digestive enzymes:** Reduce digestive work in the stomach and duodenum.

- **Mastic gum:** Binds to the lining of the stomach to help protect it.

- **Zinc carnosine:** Helps inflamed stomach lining heal.

- **Head elevation:** Sleeping with the head elevated prevents gastric juices from trickling up the esophagus.

IBS

- **Aloe:** Soothing to the stomach and intestinal lining.

- **Bitters (Angostura, Swedish):** Stimulate digestion in stomach and duodenum.

- **Enteric-coated peppermint oil:** Only get enteric-coated, otherwise, it will irritate the stomach. Helps relax the small intestine.

- **Enzymes:** Help to break down food more efficiently.

- **Magnesium citrate:** Promotes better bowel movement and is especially useful for constipation.

- **Prebiotics (inulin, beta glucan, FOS):** Basically the food to feed the probiotics in your gut. By supporting the growth of the beneficial bacteria and inhibit the growth of more harmful bacteria, you can get rid of gas and bloating.

- **Probiotics:** Higher doses of lactobacillus and bifidobacterium can reset levels of friendly intestinal flora.

- **Small, frequent meals:** Eliminates burden on the system.

CHRONIC ALLERGIES AND RESPIRATORY CONGESTION

- **Bromelain:** Mucolytic enzyme that can reduce inflammation and act as a preventive.

- **Butterbur:** Reduces inflammation in the nasal passages.

- **Essential oil such as Young Living THIEVES:** Combined with steam inhalation, these act as expectorants and decongestants. (Also germicidal.)

- **Nettles:** Natural herbal antihistamine.

- **Quercetin:** Reduces inflammation that leads to allergies and sinusitis.

ASTHMA

- **Butterbur:** Decreases inflammation and spasming.

- **Ginkgo biloba:** Helps reduce bronchial spasming.

- **Magnesium:** Relaxes muscle around the lungs. Four drops can stop acute attacks.

- **Kundalini yoga:** A type of yoga that uses breath-based techniques that serve as asthma prevention.

ECZEMA/PSORIASIS/CHRONIC DERMATITIS

- **Apple cider vinegar:** Not only applied topically, but also drank on an empty stomach when you first wake up has been proven effective to many of my clients. It takes about a month of drinking it daily to see results.

- **Evening primrose oil:** Contains GLA is a good choice for eczema.

- **Oatmeal baths:** Soothing for skin and mind.

- **Turmeric:** The active ingredient curcumin is a powerful anti-inflammatory.

- **Diet:** It is critical to do an elimination diet, especially a gluten free trial for psoriasis.

- **Meditation:** Skin conditions are highly influenced by emotions, one study showed that mindfulness meditation dramatically reduces psoriasis.

- **Scrub:** With Epsom salts and lavender oil, a scrub can soften skin, exfoliate rough patches. If you suffer with acne, psoriasis, eczema and rashes, this will also diminish the problem and calm your skin.

HEADACHES (GENERAL AND MIGRAINE)

- **Butterbur:** This herb is used for pain, upset stomach, stomach ulcers, migraine and other headaches, ongoing cough, chills, anxiety, plague, fever, trouble sleeping (insomnia), whooping cough, asthma, hay fever (allergic rhinitis), and for irritable bladder and urinary tract spasms.

- **Feverfew:** traditional herbal medicinal works well for prevention and for migraine relief.

- **Magnesium:** Deficiencies have proven to increase migraines. Magnesium also helps prevent them.

- **Riboflavin:** A vitamin B shown in some studies to prevent headaches.

- **Craniosacral therapy:** A wonderful, gentle soft touch massage technique focused on the head and neck.

- **Hard-boiled egg:** It's important to eat proteins, not carbs, as the latter would spike your blood-sugar levels and then crash, triggering more headaches. If you are not a fan of eggs, try nuts or a protein bar.

- One glass of water with a cap of apple cider vinegar and half a lemon squeezed in.

- Cold cloth over your forehead with your eyes closed.

JOINTS AND MUSCULOSKELETAL PAIN

- **Boswellia:** Ayurveda herb (AKA frankincense) that reduces joints inflammation.

- **Enzymes:** Proteolytic enzymes such as Wobenzym N and Enzymedica's Serra Gold have been shown to survive intact absorbed from the intestinal tract when taken in between meals and have a good efficacy in relieving joint pain.

- **Ginger:** Great anti inflammatory as well.

- **Glucosamine and chondroitin:** Studies show these cartilage building blocks help repair damaged cartilage.

- **Omega-3 fatty acids:** Flax or fish oil has been shown in numerous studies to reduce inflammation that causes these conditions.

- **Rhus Tox:** Oral homeopathic remedy for chronic sprains.

- **Turmeric:** Excellent general anti-inflammatory.

- **Magnets (applied to point of pain):** Studies support use in relieving discomfort. Nikken is a reliable supplier.

- **Detox bath:** Combine two cups of Epsom salts (magnesium sulfate), half a cup baking soda (alkalinizing), and 10 drops of lavender essential oil (cortisol and stress-reducing aromatherapy) to create profound relaxation and detoxification.

MOTION SICKNESS

- **Ginger:** Take 500mg of powdered or raw ginger before your flight. Ginger reduces motion sickness because stimulates receptors in the digestive track that help release the soothing hormone serotonin.

- One glass of water with a cap of apple cider vinegar and half a lemon squeezed in.

HANGOVER

- One glass of water with a cap of apple cider vinegar and half a lemon squeezed in.

- **Green juice or smoothie:** The fibers, vitamins and phytonutrients in fruits and veggies helps you burn off the alcohol and get it out of your body faster. After a night out drinking, down a 8 to 10 oz juice so you will feel better in the morning.

STINKY BREATH

Halitosis, or bad breath, is typically caused by systemic diseases, gastrointestinal and/or upper respiratory tract disorders, and microbial metabolism from your tongue, saliva or dental plaque.

- **Dentist:** A good dental clinic is usually the best place to start and address it.

- **Parsley:** A natural breath freshener. Add to your diet.

- **Chlorophyll:** In drops, add to your water as directed on the label.

- **Tongue cleaner:** A tongue cleaner is an inexpensive yet effective tool that can help curb cravings, freshen breath, and remove bacteria from the mouth. It can also help increase the power of your taste buds so you can appreciate the natural flavors of whole foods without relying on excessive salt and sugar. It is recommended that you scrape your tongue for up to 10 seconds twice a day, every day.

STRESS

- **Herbs and foods that soothe the nervous system:** Chamomile, hops, passionflower, red clover, valerian.

- **Herbs and foods for easing blood pressure:** Black cohosh, garlic, nettle, passionflower, Reishi mushrooms, Siberian ginseng, valerian.

- **Herbs and foods for relaxing before bedtime**: Catnip, chamomile, hops, lemon balm, passionflower, valerian, verbena, wild lettuce.

- **Herbal tea for insomnia:** Combine a teaspoon each of chamomile, lavender, lemon balm, passionflower and valerian to enhance your sleep.

- **Detox bath:** Combine Epsom salts (magnesium sulfate), baking soda (alkalinizing) and lavender essential oil (cortisol and stress-reducing aromatherapy) to create profound relaxation and detoxification. Here's the recipe: Fill up the bath tub with hot water and add two cups of Epsom salts, half a cup of baking soda, and 10 drops of lavender essential oil. Add one stressed human. Soak for 20 to 30 minutes. (Optional: light candles and play soothing music to enhance the experience.)

- I use this combo when I get back from a long trip as my jet lag remedy, when I am particularly sore from a workout or when I had a particularly stressful day.

- **Hot water bottle:** A hot water bottle is a great tool for creating a sense of comfort and warmth when you are sleeping. It can also be used as a warm compress for the stomach to relieve cramps and improve blood circulation to the digestive organs. On a mental and emotional level, warmth on the belly may also promote assimilation of any feelings that are left over from the day.

- **Massage:** If muscles are manually manipulated with proper pressure and understanding, the tissues will release toxins and tensions. I recommend you to find a licensed therapist to get a proper massage at least once a month. After your massages, be sure to drink plenty of water to flush out the toxins.

ENERGY

If you're coming off coffee and find you need a little something extra to help you get going in the morning, consider adding one of these natural energy boosters to your water, juice or smoothie. Use one to three teaspoons per serving (see note under matcha), adjusting for flavor and effect.

- **Cacao powder and unsweetened nibs**: The seed of the tropical cacao fruit, cacao is the primary ingredient in all chocolate and is high in antioxidants, magnesium, theobromine, and phenethylamine. The taste is bitter and chocolatey.

- **Maca powder:** Maca root is a Peruvian superfruit in the cruciferous mustard family traditionally used by indigenous cultures for energy, endurance, and libido. The powder has a sweet, nutty taste with hints of butterscotch.

- **Matcha green tea**: Matcha green tea is a finely ground, powdered, high-quality green tea from Japan known for its anticancer properties and typically used to boost metabolism and relieve stress. It is high in catechins, chlorophyll, antioxidants, and L-theanine. Matcha green tea has an intense sweetness and deeper flavor than standard grades of green tea due to its high amino acid profile. **NOTE:** Matcha is relatively high in caffeine (about 70 milligrams per teaspoon), though it does deliver L-theanine, which helps eliminate the jagged buzz. If you know you are sensitive, stick with only about a quarter or a third of a teaspoon with this one. That will give you about the amount of caffeine of a cup of green tea. (Going caffeine-free for at least the first week is optimal.)

- **Adaptogenic herbs:** Some of the best adaptogenic herbs that have been shown to boost energy and combat low energy in females and males alike include: ashwagandha, rhodiola, holy basil and ginseng.

CONSTIPATION – GAS — BLOATING

- **Hot water bottle:** A hot water bottle is a great tool for creating a sense of comfort and warmth when you are sleeping. It can also be used as a warm compress for the stomach to relieve cramps and improve blood circulation to the digestive organs. On a mental and emotional level, warmth on the belly may also promote assimilation of any feelings that are left over from the day.

- **Fiber:** Critical to the detoxification process helping to bind toxins coming into the intestines in food and then absorbing detoxified substances that come out of the gallbladder and liver. Generally 25g of daily fiber is sufficient — through a mix of soluble and insoluble fibers.

- **Aloe:** When you first wake up in the morning, have a warm glass of water with aloe juice.

ALLERGIES

- **Neti pot:** Pollution and allergens are all around you. They're in the air and can trigger allergy symptoms (such as yucky, puffy red eyes). Flush your nasal passages regularly with a neti pot daily to eliminate the side effects of air pollutants and lead to better breathing naturally.

- **Local raw unfiltered honey:** Take one spoonful a day during the pollen season to keep the symptoms at bay.

ABOUT THE AUTHOR

Eleonora is a sought-after health and wellness professional who strives to revolutionize the world of health and wellness. Motivated and inspired by a drive to contribute to the personal growth and development of the society, she incorporates the elements of health, nutrition, and personal development to encourage others in adopting a more gentle and balanced approach to life.

Born and raised in Milan, Italy, Eleonora moved to the States at the age of 21 to pursue the American dream. Her personal journey is the reason she pursued a career-change, going from marketing into integrative nutrition and qualifying in this field. Eleonora has overcome struggles, including sexual abuse, eating disorders, depression, and self-injury, then throughout years of trial and error, figured out what worked and has been sharing her method with those in need ever since.

She opened her practice in Miami in 2014, after completing her education at the Institute of Integrative Nutrition in New York. Since then, she has been coaching women all over the world helping them improve their health and relationship between their body and food, along with permanent weight loss through implementing a few simple diet and lifestyle changes. She has been selected to work with a number of renowned brands such as Victoria Beckham's team, Radio Health UK and WeWork to promote health and wellness.

Her approach to nutrition is different from what else is out there, as it was built on personal experience with eating disorders, and years of helping other women improve their relationship with their body and food.

Eleonora's method incorporates health, nutrition and personal development as part of her personalized plans, making it uniquely comprehensive – there are few programs in the world that take this approach, and even fewer with long-lasting results. Eleonora believes that your emotions play just as much a role in your wellbeing as food does, and that in order to make any lasting change in your life and eating habits you need to address your emotions.

You can stay up to date with her by visiting her website: www.eleonoracbastos.com or follow her on Instagram @eleonoracbastos.

DISCLAIMER (Continued)

Eleonora Calcada Bastos (the author) is not a licensed medical care provider, healthcare professional, medical doctor, therapist, psychiatrist, clinical psychologist, or licensed counselor, nor does she practice medicine, and represents that she has no expertise in diagnosing, examining, or treating medical conditions of any kind, or in determining the effect of any specific statement on a medical condition.

As such, neither the publisher nor the author shall be liable for any physical, psychological, emotional, financial, or commercial damages, including, but not limited to, special, incidental, consequential or other damages. Furthermore, the publisher and author are not responsible for any specific health or allergy needs that may require medical supervision and are not liable for any damages or negative consequences from any application, treatment, action or preparation, to any person reading or following the information in this book.

It is imperative that you consult your physician before using this product or starting any program, as fitness training and diet can result in serious or fatal injury. If you engage in this program, you agree that you do it at your own risk, are voluntarily participating in these activities, assume all risk of injury to yourself, and agree to release and discharge Eleonora Calcada Bastos from any and all claims or causes of action, known or unknown, arising out of Eleonora Calcada Bastos negligence.

If you have a health problem, medical emergency, or a general health question, we always recommend you consult your doctor.

All books provided by Eleonora Calcada Bastos are on an "as is" and "as available" basis. Thus, all purchasers and/or readers of any Eleonora Calcada Bastos handouts, e-books, written material, whether provided in hardcopy or digitally (together 'Material') expressly agree that their download, use, application or interpretation is done at their sole and exclusive risk. To the full extent permissible by applicable Federal and State law, Eleonora Calcada Bastos disclaims all warranties, express or implied, including, but not limited to, implied warranties or merchantability. Eleonora Calcada Bastos does not warrant that any digital material will be free of viruses or other harmful components. Eleonora Calcada Bastos shall not be liable for any damages of any kind arising from the download, use, application or interpretation of any Eleonora Calcada Bastos material, including, but not limited to direct, indirect, incidental, punitive, and consequential damages.

RESOURCES

Jamieson, Alex (2006-06-27). The Great American Detox Diet: Feel Better, Look Better, and Lose Weight by Cleaning Up Your Diet (Kindle Locations 2061-2062). Rodale. Kindle Edition.

Merrell, Woodson; Beth Augustine, Mary; Dodle, Hillari (2013-12-24). The Detox Prescription: Supercharge Your Health, Strip Away Pounds, and Eliminate the Toxins Within (Kindle Locations 6104-6114). Rodale Books. Kindle Edition.

Hyman, Mark (2014-02-25). The Blood Sugar Solution 10-Day Detox Diet: Activate Your Body's Natural Ability to Burn Fat and Lose Weight Fast (p81). Little, Brown and Company. Kindle Edition.

www.mindbodygreen.com

www.Mercola.com

www.draxe.com

Kris Carr

Marie Forleo

Rosenthal, Joshua (2015-04-22). The Power of Primary Food: Nourishment Beyond The Plate (Kindle Locations 245-257). Integrative Nutrition. Kindle Edition.

Women's Health

http://www.whatsonmyfood.org/food.jsp?food=WR

http://natureworksbest.com/naturopathy-works/food-cravings/ (Craving chart)

http://www.organicauthority.com/the-top-10-most-inflammatory-foods-in-the-american-diet/

http://www.arizonaadvancedmedicine.com/Articles/2013/June/Inflammation-A-Common-Denominator-of-Disease.aspx

http://fructosemalabsorptionhq.com/fructose-malabsorption-guide

http://www.greenmedinfo.com/page/dark-side-wheat-new-perspectives-celiac-disease-wheat-intolerance-sayer-ji

http://amymyersmd.com

FOOTNOTES

[i] https://www.ncbi.nlm.nih.gov/books/NBK493173/

[ii] http://www.glamour.com/story/shocking-body-image-news-97-percent-of-women-will-be-cruel-to-their-bodies-today

[iii] https://www.consumerreports.org/heart-disease/take-charge-of-your-heart-health/

[iv] http://www.onlinejacc.org/content/70/20/2519?sso=1&sso_redirect_count=1&access_token=

[v] http://www.ncbi.nlm.nih.gov/pmc/articles/PMC4473616/

[vi] http://www.greenmedinfo.com/page/dark-side-wheat-new-perspectives-celiac-disease-wheat-intolerance-sayer-ji

[vii] UNEP and OECD, 2,6-di-tert-butyl-p-cresol (BHT) Screening Information Data Set: Initial Assessment Report (Paris: OECD, 2002), http://www.inchem.org/documents/sids/sids/128370.pdf.

[viii] Baur, A.K. et al., "The lung tumor promoter, butylated hydroxytoluene (BHT), causes chronic inflammation in promotion-sensitive BALB/cByJ mice but not in promotion-resistant CXB4 mice," Toxicology 169, no. 1 (December 2001): 1-15.

[ix] http://wsm.wsu.edu/s/index.php?id=749

[x] http://pubs.acs.org/didi/abs/10.1021/jf030217n?journalCode=jafcau

[xi] http://www.ewg.org/research/shoppers-guide-to-avoiding-gmos

[xii] http://authoritynutrition.com/how-much-protein-per-day/

[xiii] UCLA Health System May 15, 2012

[xiv] http://fructosemalabsorptionhq.com/fructose-malabsorption-guide

[xv] http://www.rodalesorganiclife.com/food/trying-lose-weight-stay-away-artificial-sweeteners

[xvi] http://www.cancer.gov/cancertopics/factsheet/Risk/artificial-sweeteners

[xvii] http://articles.mercola.com/sites/articles/archive/2001/02/28/obesity-soft-drinks.aspx

[xviii] http://www.consumerreports.org/cro/magazine/2015/01/will-a-gluten-free-diet-really-make-you-healthier/index.html

[xix] http://www.ncbi.nlm.nih.gov/pmc/articles/PMC4488826/

[xx] http://www.ncbi.nlm.nih.gov/pubmed/26043918

[xx] Adaptogenic Herbs: Nature's Solution To Stress By Edward C. Wallace, N.D., D.C. — https://chiro.org/nutrition/FULL/Adaptogenic_Herbs.shtml April 5th 2019

[xxi] Mindful August 27, 2012 and Globe and Mail August 24, 2012

[xxii] http://www.who.int/trade/glossary/story073/en/

Printed in Poland
by Amazon Fulfillment
Poland Sp. z o.o., Wrocław

55483998R10201